NOTIFY IN 7

Written By

JANET GREENWALD

&

LAURA GREENWALD

Published by Stuf Productions/Lion And The Rock Entertainment

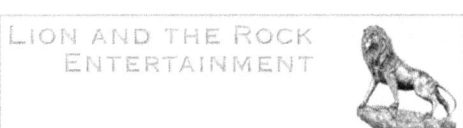

Manufactured in the United States of America

ISBN: 978-1505373042

BEFORE YOU BEGIN

Welcome to Notify In 7!

Notify In 7 is filled with all of the tools you and your staff need to perform next of kin notifications and patient identification quickly and easily while enhancing communication and patient satisfaction.

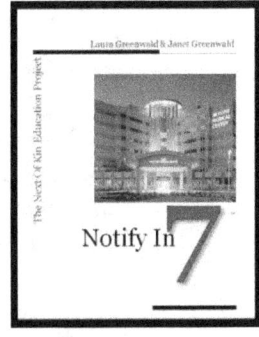

It's actually three books in one.

Notify In 7

How To Locate An ICE Contact On Your Patient's Smartphone

The Notify In 7 Training Manual

All three sections work together to give you everything you need to roll out the Seven Steps System facility-wide.

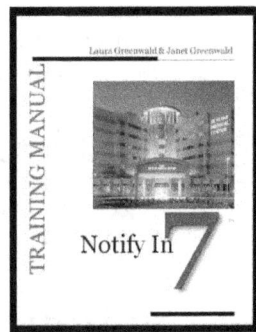

The book also includes downloadable patient tracking workflows, tools and training materials that will provide your Emergency Department staff, managers and Risk Management professionals with comprehensive training, while giving you and your hospital a fully operational Next of Kin Notification System in just 90 days.

But before you can get started, you'll need to go and download the materials that come with the book. Just go to www.nokep.org/notifyin7dwnld.htm and register with the special code NI72015 to confirm that you're a book owner.

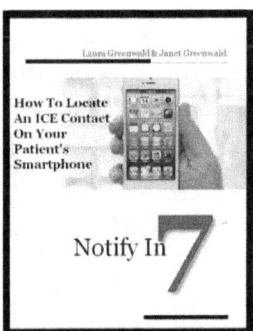

contents

introduction

the seven steps

patient care tools

Published By

The Next of Kin Education Project
www.getyourstufftogether.com
webmaster1@nokep.org

© Stuf Productions 2014

patient care tools cont'd

reducing liability

introduction

REDUCING LIABILITY
Simple steps your facility can take to avoid liability while increasing patient care & safety

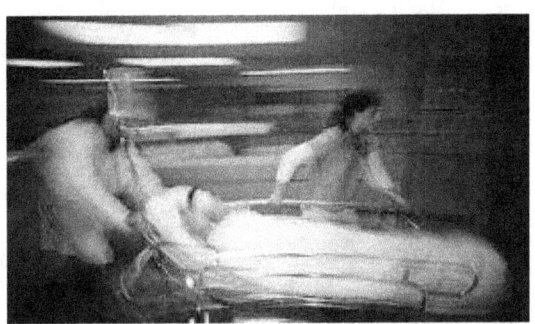

> Despite having her daughter's contact information right on her chart, the hospital failed to notify her family that she'd been hospitalized, for six days, just hours before she died...

The screech of tires on wet pavement. The crushing pain of a massive MI. Being caught in the wrong place at the tragically wrong time. Suddenly, instead of being part of the team of caregivers, you're the one on the gurney looking into the unfamiliar faces of a trauma team who knows nothing about you or your medical history.

In the blink of an eye, anyone can find himself in need of emergency care. In California alone, nearly ten million people require emergency room care every year, and of those, one and a half million arrive in critical condition.

That's exactly what happened to Elaine Sullivan. A very active 71 year old woman, Elaine fell at home while getting into the bathtub. When paramedics arrived, they realized that injuries to her mouth and head had made her unable to communicate, or as the hospital later discovered, to give informed consent for her own care.

Although stable for the first few days, she began to slip into critical condition. On the seventh day, Elaine died. But that tragedy was soon overshadowed by another. Despite having her daughter's contact information clearly indicated on the front of her chart, the hospital failed to notify her family that she'd been hospitalized until six days later. Finally the call was made hours before she died, unnecessarily alone.

Elaine Sullivan was my mother.

When my daughter Laura and I found out how long she had actually been hospitalized, our grief turned to action. We began to hear similar stories from around the country, circumstances where people who had been injured in accidents or had fallen ill at home, and were hospitalized for hours, days or in some cases a week, without so much as a phone call to the patient's spouse, family or emergency contact.

Medical professionals nationwide agree that timely next of kin notification is vital. Not only is it important to have a family member present to comfort the patient, but to make informed decisions the patient can't make for himself and to provide the medical history that could very well make the difference between life and death. Although most hospitals notify the next of kin of unconscious ED arrivals relatively quickly, it's extremely easy for staffers to get busy or distracted enough, to forget to make that call in a timely fashion. In my mother's case that simple act would have saved her life. Not only would we have been able to know that she'd been hospitalized and had the time to fly back to Chicago to be there with her, but we would have been able to make sure that she received the care she needed, and to give the physicians treating her, the medical and prescription drug history that would have prevented the drug interactions and complications that were responsible for her death.

Even though prompt notification is an important part of outstanding patient care, we discovered only a handful of states have regulations that mandate notifications within a specific time frame, if at all. So we partnered with legislators in California and Illinois to create The Next of Kin Law. Recently enacted, the law simply states that a hospital must make reasonable efforts, (outlined in a simple checklist), to contact the next of kin of patients who come into a hospital unconscious or physically unable to give informed consent, within 24 hours of their admission. To date, six states have NOK statutes and a federal version is being considered in Congress.

As soon as the two laws were enacted, hospitals across the country started hearing about our story and began asking for simple, concrete ways to perform NOK notifications quickly and easily – ways to keep those kinds of tragedies from happening in their own facilities.

To answer that need, we worked with medical professionals nationwide, to create the Seven Steps System. Notify In 7 and the Notify In 7 Training Program is a comprehensive guide to creating a notification program in your own facility. Whether your own internal notification procedures need a bit of streamlining, or if you need to start from scratch, this guide uses a **Six Sigma** approach to giving hospitals the background and tools they need to:

Evaluate trauma patient's next of kin status and needs

• Make next of kin notifications quickly and easily in every situation.

• Identify and treat John/Jane Does

• Includes work flows and patient chart worksheets to track patients and document steps taken to reduce liability.

It provides everything you need to evaluate current notification procedures, design, create and execute a facility-wide notification program.

Creating a Program also includes, tools your staff can use on the patient care floor and Seven Steps Patient Chart Worksheets, that you can use as part of your own charting system.

The full program has been created to be used as a training tool and a reference guide for all of the departments within your facility that deal with or set policy for the care of emergent patients, including the Chief of Trauma and the Emergency Department, the Chief of Nursing, Chief of Staff, your Risk Management team, your Social Workers, Compliance Officer and even your CIO and marketing staff.

Are you ready to learn more about the Seven Steps System?

Great, then let's get started! §

Benefits to Using the Seven Steps

Reduces hospital and physician liability by bringing in a decision maker, (the patient's next of kin or surrogate decision maker), while the patient is unable to make his own health care decisions.

Promotes good will, portrays your hospital as even more of a caring, family-friendly institution.

Provides a simple continuum of care that every hospital both large and small can use, to simplify system-wide protocols and training.

Patient care and satisfaction increase, mortality and liability decrease.

Increases effectiveness in treating different segments of your community.

Increases effectiveness of risk management.

Increases effectiveness of social service.

Decreases workload of nursing staff by naming clear-cut, next of kin notification responsibilities and departments to which notifications must be referred.

Easy to use training and reminder materials to bring staff and department heads up to speed quickly. In states with next of kin statutes, eliminates liability of unknowingly failing to comply with the Next of Kin Law.

Provides ways to safeguard your own family and friends, in the event of an emergency.

Makes staff's work easier by giving them the information they need to locate a patient's medical history and treat him with his history in mind, eliminating the learning curve of treating an unknown person.

WHY WE NEED THIS INFORMATION

How important is a patient's family to his recovery? More important that we first thought...

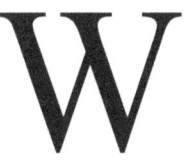

When I trained in medical school, hospitals were considered private places where a patient turned over his/her body and mind to the ministrations of doctors and nurses. Family was really kept at a distance. Visiting hours were tightly controlled. The people who were an integral part of the patient's life were allowed entry for only a brief time. They had no place in the care of the patient.

Times have changed. My own personal journey with this change happened a decade ago. One of my nurses told me about an article in the nursing literature about allowing family to be present during resuscitation efforts. As an emergency physician, I was intrigued by this idea. We already had a liberal policy of allowing family to stay with our patients in their rooms, but how would it work to have outsiders watch as we furiously raced to restart a stopped heart, to slide a tube into a collapsed vein in order to give life-renewing medications? Would the family faint, try to stop us, throw themselves across the bed?

Although it was radical at the time, we decided to try it out. In order to minimize the chance of a fainting relative, we created a very controlled environment where the family would be oriented to what they would see and hear before they were brought back to the room. I remember the first woman who was brought back to the treatment room where I was trying to restart her father's heart. She entered the room, looked around and blurted, "It's just like on TV!" At the time, I was startled. Upon reflection, I realized television has unshrouded the mysteries of medicine for many. Our concerns were unnecessary.

That woman was the first of many daughters, of many sons, brothers, sisters, wives, husbands, mothers and fathers we allowed, no—not allowed—invited into our emergency rooms to be with loved ones. The families told us they gained comfort from being with the patient. They could see we were bringing all of our skill and energy to cure, to heal. But we gained, too.

The family was able to participate. They were able to bring the force of their love to help the patient. They could also give us information. I can't count the times these families saved us precious minutes by adding information on health status, past history and current medications that speeded our diagnosis and treatments.

When a story about our emergency department aired on national television, I received a call from Laura Greenwald in California. Her grandmother had died—alone—in a Chicago hospital without family having been called. Laura and her mother Janet were determined to see that such an omission would not happen to other patients and their families. If you are reading this, it is because of the Greenwald's efforts. It is because they and I want you to know that the patient should not be isolated.

Just as doctors, nurses, technicians, pharmacist, dietitians and many others make up a team to improve the health of the patients in their care, family and friends can play an important part in contributing to the patient's well being. As a medical professional, you are a diagnostician, a caregiver and a healer. But most of all, you are the patient's advocate. And so is his family. This kit contains information that will show you how your patient's family can be an effective part of their loved one's health care team. §

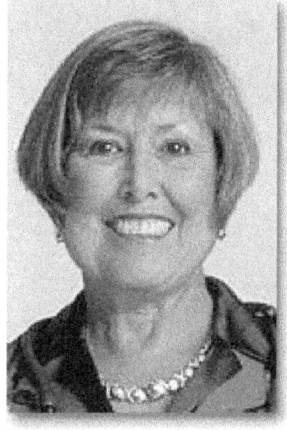

Nancy J. Auer, MD, FACEP

Past President, American College of Emergency Physicians

Vice President for Medical Affairs

Swedish Health Systems

Seattle, Washington

the seven steps

ONE STEP AT A TIME

How to provide better patient care and reduce unnecessary liability, in one simple system

The Seven Steps to Successful Notification is an easy-to-use system based on tools successfully used by hospitals nationwide. It provides your hospital staff with all of the steps necessary to:

• Identify and locate your unconscious patient's next of kin or surrogate decision maker.

• Improve patient care by locating your patient's medical history, personal physician, and insurance information.

• Provide the facility with documentation of the steps taken to find the patient's next of kin, to make the notification, and identify the staff members responsible for making it, thereby releasing you from subsequent liability.

• In states with statutes requiring next of kin notifications within a certain amount of time, provides proof that the facility has met its statutory responsibility.

1. Confirm Patient Status

2. Examine personal effects for emergency contacts

3. Locate patient's home number

4. Seek other sources for contact information

5. Make the notification call

6. Recall main contact or second phone number

7. Shift to Follow Up

The Seven Steps

In the documents that you downloaded, along with other tools, you received a Patient Tracking Worksheet and Patient Tracking Chart Page that you can use to track your ED patients through the notification process. This section will show you how to use it.

Let's watch the Seven Steps in action, through the eyes of the nurse manager of Care Central's Trauma Unit, Carolee Cummins.

Carolee comes on duty this morning just as a hit and run is pulling up at the emergency bay. She meets the gurney and runs along side, paying rapt attention to the paramedic's bullet, while she and her team do their own evaluation. The paramedic's last comment stops her cold. This pretty thirtyish, woman who is in grave danger of bleeding out, has no identification on her. Carolee starts a chart for her patient and turns her attention back to the trauma.

Step One

Step 1 Confirm Patient Status

Is patient unconscious? ___Yes ___No

If the patient is conscious, is he/she physically or mentally unable to give informed consent. ___Yes ___No
Does the patient have a family member or surrogate decision maker in attendance? ___Yes ___No
If the answers to all three of these questions are yes, page **The Notifier** on duty and have them continue with **Step 2**.

When a patient like this comes in, Carolee is glad that she and her team use the Seven Steps System. The triage nurse who usually performs the role of **Assessor**, the team member who assesses the patient's next of kin needs, is busy right now, so Carolee takes over. She grabs a Patient Tracking Worksheet and begins the notification process right in the trauma room, by answering the first question.

Is the patient unconscious or if conscious, physically unable to give informed consent?

After the team confirms that the patient is unresponsive to everything but deep pain, Carolee checks "yes".

Does the patient have a family member or surrogate decision maker in attendance?

Carolee asks one of the aides to check the waiting room to see if any family members came in with their patient. "No", the aide confirms, "she came in alone". Again Carolee checks yes, and the notification process begins.

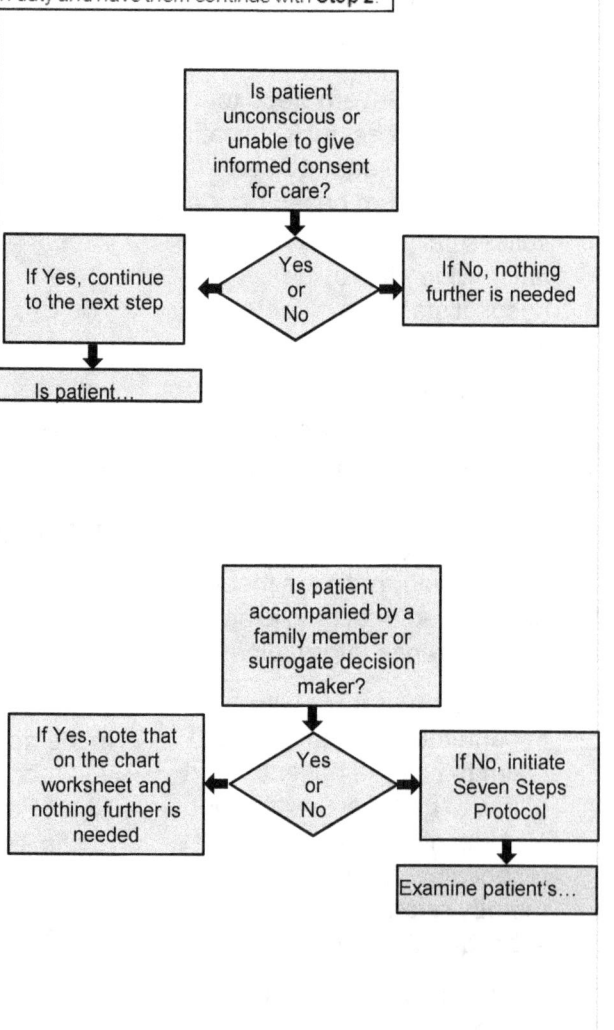

Step Two

Step 2 **Examine personal effects for emergency contacts**
Examine patient's personal effects for an emergency contact number. If patient doesn't have an emergency card in his/her wallet, check the patient's purse, brief case or day planner, clothing, or cell phone for home or emergency numbers.
Was an emergency contact name found? ___Yes ___No _____Time   If yes, go to step 5. If no, go to **step 3**.

When Care Central began to use the Seven Steps System, they appointed Carolee as Trauma Notification Manager, the team member who oversees next of kin notifications in the ED.

Since she already feels invested in this patient, Carolee puts on her **Notifier** cap and begins step two of the process. The Notifier is the team member who searches for the patient's emergency contact information or in this case, identity and when found, makes the actual notification.

Examine patient's personal effects for an emergency contact number. If he/she doesn't have an emergency card in his/her wallet, check the patient's purse, briefcase, clothing, or cell phone for home or emergency numbers.

Examine patient's personal effects for an emergency contact number. Was an emergency contact number found?

Note that no number was found. Try to locate the patient's home telephone number. Was a home number found?

Yes or No

Place a call to make the notification, and record the details on the chart. This includes the time the cal was made, the name and phone number of that contact and any others found (relationship, field to record result of call) Is the contact on the way to the hospital?

Carolee looks for the young woman's emergency contact numbers or clues to those numbers, by examining her personal effects. Most of the time, Carolee finds the emergency information quite easily, right in her patient's wallet, on a driver's license, emergency contact cards, insurance cards or personal phone books.

In this case her search takes only a moment – the only thing this woman had with her were her house keys. If she had a wallet or a purse, it was destroyed in the accident.

Carolee goes through the pockets of her patient's jogging shorts and finds one small clue to her identity – a few message blanks from work that she must have stuffed in her pocket to take care of later. They're all made out to Katherine McCauley. Progress!

If Step 2 had turned up nothing and her patient had still been a Jane Doe, Carolee would have skipped down to Step 7, involving her **Follow Up** person or Social Services in her search. But since Carolee's patient now has a name, she goes directly to Step 3.

Step Three

Step 3 Locate patient's home number
If you can't find a specific person/number named as an emergency contact, try to locate the patient's home telephone number.
Home number found? ___ Yes ___ No ___ Time _____ If yes, go to step 5. If no, go to **step 4**.

Now Carolee will have to get a bit more creative.

As Katherine found out the hard way, life can present major challenges for patients, not to mention an emergency department staff. A quick run to the store without taking your ID, interrupted by a sudden accident or heart attack, can put even the most conscientious person into jeopardy. In upcoming sections of this Program, you'll find more ways to find a patient's contact information quickly and easily.

If you can't find a specific person/number specified as an emergency contact, try to locate the patient's home telephone number.

Usually Carolee would go through her mental checklist of ways she's found patient's home phone numbers in the past: checking the speed dial of a patient's cell phone for numbers labeled "home" or "work"; the contact pages of a Filofax, or the address book of a PDA. Even a briefcase can contain a patient's business card, or a company letterhead on documents.

If Carolee had found a home number or an emergency contact on any of these items, she would have gone right to Step 5. Since Katherine has none of these things with her, Carolee documents that fact on the worksheet along with the time, and proceeds to Step 4.

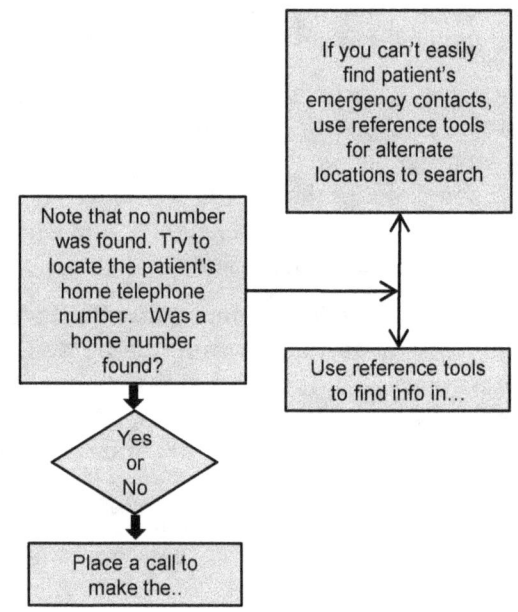

Step Four

	Step 4 Seek other sources for contact information
	Look for the patient's emergency contact information on records from his/her previous hospital admissions, or by calling his doctor's office or his insurance company.

Was an emergency contact found? ___Yes ___No _____Time   If yes, go to **step 5**. If no, go to step 7.

Carolee almost never gets to this section, but when she does, she knows it's time to crank her investigative skills into high gear! Since she knows her patient's name, her next step will take her to the hospital's medical records department.

Look for the patient's emergency contact information on records from his/her previous hospital admissions, or by calling his doctor's office or insurance company.

Chances are, if Katherine lives in the area, this isn't her first visit to Care Central. Even if the old records don't include the patient's next of kin or surrogate decision maker, Carolee will be able to get it, by phoning Katherine's home number, physician or insurer.

If Carolee still hadn't been able to find information on her patient, she would have gone directly to Step 7 and turned the Patient Tracking Worksheet over to the **Follow Up**, the team member, usually from Social Service or Patient Advocacy, who handles more complex notifications.

But Carolee quickly locates Katherine's name on a chart from last year when she was admitted for the birth of her son. Success!

Now on to Step 5.

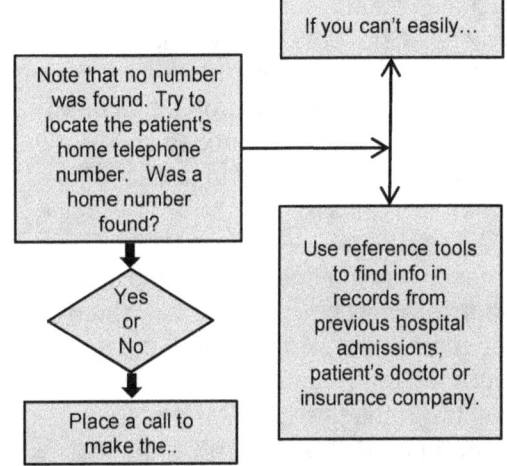

	Step 5 Make the notification call

When a contact has been identified from step 2, 3, or 4, place the phone call to make the notification.

Call made to (contact's name, relationship to the patient & number):

Note the results of the call:

Is contact coming to the hospital? ___Yes ___No
If yes, this section is complete. _____ Initial _____ Time   If there was no answer, or if you had to leave a message, go to **step 6**

Since Carolee's first priority is notifying the patient's next of kin or surrogate decision maker, her aim is to contact the right person as soon as possible. She is disappointed to hear Katherine's answering machine pick up. Carolee hates doing a notification this way. She leaves a message for Katherine's husband, hoping that he'll pick it up quickly. Many times the only person Carolee has been able to reach is a relative or friend, so she is always careful to document the name and relationship of any person she talks to.

Occasionally the only information she finds is the patient's family physician or insurance company. In that case she makes sure that the doctor's office or insurance representative knows that she needs to speak with the family ASAP and then follows up within an hour or so. Carolee has learned the hard way, never to assume that a third party is going to take care of a notification. Since Care Central is the facility treating the patient and is the one in need of medical history to give Katherine the best care possible, it's Care Central's responsibility to make sure the notification takes place.

Even though Care Central's responsibility is technically met the moment Carolee left the message for Katherine's husband, the hospital has made it a priority to follow up with another phone call if a patient's next of kin doesn't arrive or return the hospital's call within the next two hours.

She documents the results on the Worksheet, initials that the section is complete and notes the time that the call occurred.

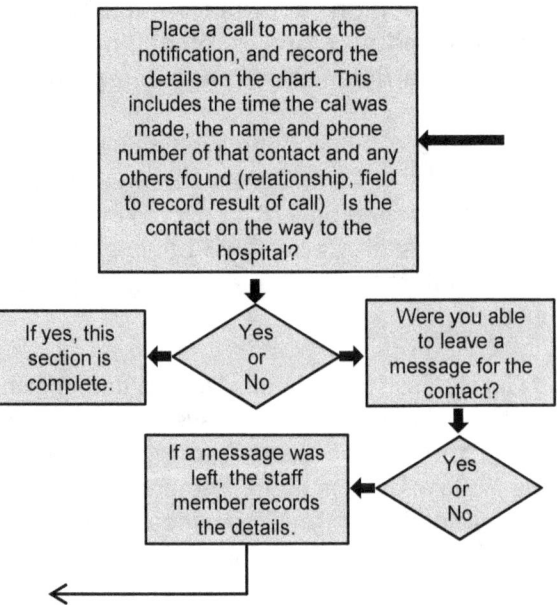

The entire process has taken Carolee less than ten minutes, and by using Care Central's Patient Tracking Worksheet, Carolee's hospital now has a documented account of her efforts. If her patient or her patient's family were ever to question the fact that notification was attempted or the steps that were taken, the hospital will be able to prove that procedure was properly followed.

Step Six

Step 6 Recall main contact or second phone number
If you left a message with the emergency contact or patient's home number, but the person called hasn't come into the hospital or called back within two hours, call again to leave one more message (see step 5).
If you have found a second contact number, call it as well.
Second call made to (contact's name, relationship to the patient & number):   Note the results of the call:
Is contact coming to the hospital? ___Yes ___No   If yes, this section is complete. _____ Initial _____ Time   If there was no answer, or if you had to leave a message, page the   **Follow Up** team member on duty to continue with **step 7**. Name of **Follow Up**: _____ Title:

Answering machines and voice mail are wonderful and no one can imagine life without them – unless it's an emergency and you can't get a hold of the person you need to speak with!

Two hours later, the husband still hasn't arrived and Katherine's condition is worsening.   Doctors are wondering if she has an undetermined, underlying condition that is keeping her BP from stabilizing despite their efforts. Carolee quickly proceeds to Step 6.

Recall main contact or second phone number.

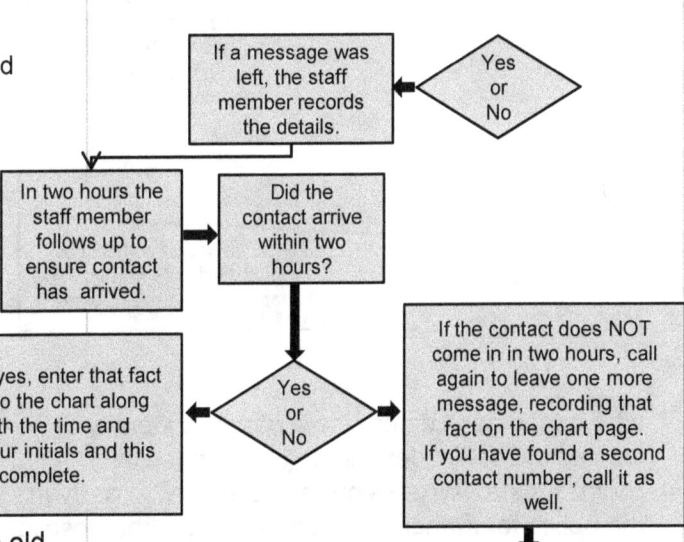

Carolee found Katherine's work number on the old chart, but before she tries it, she tries the home number one more time. Katherine's husband Scott answers. Only minutes before, he'd forgotten an important brief and ran back home to get it, allowing him to pick up Carolee's message. A short while later, he arrives at the hospital and fills the trauma team in on his wife's medical history. Changes in her treatment are immediately made and hours later, Katherine, now alert and stable, is on her way to a full recovery.

Had Carolee not been able to reach anyone at Katherine's home, she would have called the second number, then documented the results on the Worksheet, with the time and her initials.

If she still hadn't been able to reach anyone in person or if the relative hadn't shown up at the facility, she would have noted that on the Worksheet and paged her **Follow Up** person to proceed with Step 7.

Step Seven

	Step 7 Shift to Follow Up

If no contact name or number was found by performing steps 2 through 4, or if you haven't been able to speak directly to the contact identified, give the information you've identified to your social service department or department/person specified by your facility's policy, for further research.

Gave information to: (name & department)

At _____ (time) by _____ (your name) _____ (status) _____ (initials).

Every once in a while, despite Carolee's best efforts, she has to shift the notification to her Follow Up person.

```
If the contact does NOT
come in in two hours, call
again to leave one more
message, recording that
fact on the chart page.
If you have found a
second contact number,
call it as well.
```

```
In two hours the staff member
follows up to ensure contact
has arrived. If contact has
not arrived note that on the
chart and go to the next step.
```

```
Yes
or
No
```

```
Use reference
tools to find
contact info or
identify patients
in unusual
situations.
```

```
If no contact name or number has
been located for patient or if you
have not been able to speak
directly to the emergency contact,
send the information gathered, to
Follow Up.   The Seven Steps
Protocol is complete.
```

If he or she can't determine a patient's identity or locate next of kin, depending on the hospital's policies, the case goes on to social service or even the police for further research. Although the hospital has met its legal responsibility to take reasonable efforts to notify the patient's next of kin, the patient still needs intervention.

By shifting the notification process over to her Follow Up team member, Carolee is confident that everything possible will be done to find her patient's family. In upcoming sections, you'll find tips and tools to help you deal with identifying Jane/John Does and handling the effort quickly and easily.

On the following page you'll find a copy of the Patient Tracking Worksheet using the Seven Steps System.

Sample Patient Tracking Worksheet

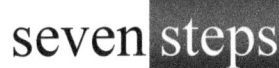

seven steps

SEVEN STEPS TO SUCCESSFUL NOTIFICATION	PATIENT TRACKING WORKSHEET

Patient Name:	Date:	Time Admitted to ED:

Name of **Assessor**:	Title:	Name of **Notifier**:	Title:

Step 1 Confirm Patient Status

Is patient unconscious? ___Yes ___No

If the patient is conscious, is he/she physically or mentally unable to give informed consent. ___Yes ___No
Does the patient have a family member or surrogate decision maker in attendance? ___Yes ___No
If the answers to all three of these questions are yes, page **The Notifier** on duty and have them continue with **Step 2**.

Step 2 Examine personal effects for emergency contacts

Examine patient's personal effects for an emergency contact number. If patient doesn't have an emergency card in his/her wallet, check the patient's purse, brief case or day planner, clothing, or cell phone for home or emergency numbers.

Was an emergency contact name found? ___Yes ___No _____Time   If yes, go to step 5. If no, go to **step 3**.

Step 3 Locate patient's home number

If you can't find a specific person/number named as an emergency contact, try to locate the patient's home telephone number.

Home number found? ___Yes ___No _____Time   If yes, go to step 5. If no, go to **step 4**.

Step 4 Seek other sources for contact information

Look for the patient's emergency contact information on records from his/her previous hospital admissions, or by calling his doctor's office or his insurance company.

Was an emergency contact found? ___Yes ___No _____Time   If yes, go to **step 5**. If no, go to step 7.

Step 5 Make the notification call

When a contact has been identified from step 2, 3, or 4, place the phone call to make the notification.

Call made to (contact's name, relationship to the patient & number):

Note the results of the call:

Is contact coming to the hospital? ___Yes ___No
If yes, this section is complete. _____ Initial _____ Time   If there was no answer, or if you had to leave a message, go to **step 6**.

Step 6 Recall main contact or second phone number

If you left a message with the emergency contact or patient's home number, but the person called hasn't come into the hospital or called back within two hours, call again to leave one more message (see step 5).

If you have found a second contact number, call it as well.

Second call made to (contact's name, relationship to the patient & number):
Note the results of the call:

Is contact coming to the hospital? ___Yes ___No
If yes, this section is complete. _____ Initial _____ Time   If there was no answer, or if you had to leave a message, page the
Follow Up team member on duty to continue with **step 7**. Name of **Follow Up**:   Title:

Step 7 Shift to Follow Up

If no contact name or number was found by performing steps 2 through 4, or if you haven't been able to speak directly to the contact identified, give the information you've identified to your social service department or department/person specified by your facility's policy, for further research.

Gave information to: (name & department)

At _____ (time) by _____ (your name) _____ (status) _____ (initials).

ALL IN A DAY'S WORK

Next of kin notifications from the nurses' perspective

After being hit by a car in a crosswalk, a young man in his twenties arrived in our emergency department in critical condition, with a severe head injury. I'm the trauma director at a bustling city trauma center and this was exactly the type of patient that I hate to see come in. He had absolutely nothing with him to identify him. The only clue to his identity was the location where the accident occurred, a busy city intersection. It was a hectic day in our ED and as patient after patient came through the doors, my staff and I kept telling ourselves that we would get down to the task of looking for the young man's name and family as soon as our staff nurses had a few moments. After all, he was receiving the best care possible and that was the most important thing – wasn't it?

The next morning, I began to wonder what became of our patient, who was now resting in the ICU. I went up to see him the first chance I got and when I looked at the still unconscious man's chart, I couldn't believe what I was seeing. No one had even begun to initiate a search. I immediately tossed everything else aside and tried to find clues to this man's identity. By the end of the day, I had exhausted all of my resources. Nothing. My John Doe wasn't doing well, in fact things were touch and go and I knew I'd have to do something quickly.

So I began with what I had – a physical description – which was difficult with the cranial and facial swelling. Asian male, dark hair, round face... I opened his eyes – which were a rich, warm brown. Knowing that he was lying in that bed alone, his family – if he had one – without a clue that he'd been critically injured, overwhelmed me. I sent the description over to the police, who began to canvass the area.

A day later, the police still hadn't received any leads. In the meantime John Doe's condition worsened.

I went up to the unit and decided to search through my patient's clothes one more time. In the last pocket, I felt a piece of paper – a dog-eared business card for a grocery store a few blocks away from the intersection where the accident had occurred. I dialed the number and reached the owner of the store who had frantically been helping my patient's mother search for him. To ensure I had the right person, I asked him a few questions. "He's an Asian man, dark hair." "No," the grocer stopped me – "the boy we're looking for isn't Asian, he's Caucasian and he has Down's Syndrome". I looked down at the patient. He was so swollen, that his eyes could easily been mistaken for being slanted, but on closer examination, the signs were unmistakable, my patient had Down's. That's what kept the police from realizing that my John Doe was their missing person.

He worked bagging groceries at the little store every day after school. He was on his way home when a car veered into the crosswalk, striking him just a few blocks from his house. My patient – Peter. Now he not only had a name, he had a family who rushed to his side. Despite the fact that he received the best care available, Peter died the next day, his mother at his bedside. Although my team and I were relieved we found his family in time, I felt horrible that two of his final three days were spent alone. And so did his mother. She stopped by to see me after her son had passed away and accepted my profuse apologies. Gracefully, I thought, considering what I might have done and said, had our situations been reversed.

Before she left, Peter's mom looked me squarely in the eye. "You took wonderful care of my son physically and for that, I'll always be grateful. As for not finding me right away, I won't take that any further, as long as you promise me one thing. Every time a John Doe comes into this emergency room from now on, I want you to think about Peter and I want you to make sure that you do everything you can do, as soon as possible to bring that patient's family to his bedside."

I kept my promise. Thanks to Peter, a month later we not only had a brand new policy regarding John Does, but we had a system in place to handle next of kin notifications and a straightforward line of responsibility for performing them. Now when an unconscious patient comes into our ED everyone on our staff knows exactly what to do. §

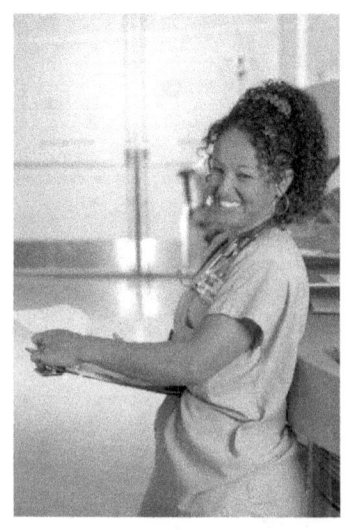

FACILITATING COMMUNICATION

Just a few simple steps to help communication-impaired patients, can make a huge impact in their hospital stay. It might even save their lives.

We've all seen patients who were far beyond the reach of medical treatment suddenly defy the odds and recover. We've also seen patients who were well on the road to recovery, take a turn for the worse for seemingly no reason at all. No matter what the technology or how terrific we are at our jobs, sometimes medicine just isn't enough.

Case in point, a few years ago, my Grandma, in her mid-sixties at the time, had a moderate CVA. No matter what her doctors did for her, she wasn't regaining consciousness, defying explanation. My mom and I were living and working in Los Angeles and Grandma was two thousand miles away in Chicago. When the doctor called to tell us about the stroke, he not only said that Grandma might not live through the night, but that she might not last the few hours it would take us to fly to her side.

Mom and I both felt very strongly that we had to talk to her for what might be the last time, before we got on the plane. Hearing our voices and knowing that someone was with her, had always made a huge difference in any difficulty she faced.

So Mom got the head nurse on the phone and asked if she could get a phone to Grandma. Asking quickly turned to pleading – we needed to tell Grandma to hold on and that we were coming. The nurse basically dismissed the notion – what possible good could THAT do? It took a while, but Mom finally convinced the nurse to put a phone up to Grandma's ear.

We were able to tell her how much we loved her, that she was going to be fine and that we were on our way. By the time the nurse came back on the phone, she was speechless. Evidently the moment Grandma heard our voices her eyelids began to flutter. Her vitals stabilized, her eyes opened for the first time since she'd been in the hospital and she looked straight up at the nurse and then around the room looking for us. Two weeks later, she was out of the hospital and on her way to rehab.

That's the miracle of communication.

Whether it's a family member, a friend or just a familiar face, patients need to have the people they love surrounding them, when they're ill, in pain, or afraid. As caregivers, it's part of the job to realize that patients might be too ill or physically unable to initiate the contact they so desperately need, on their own.

I wish that were the end of the story. A few years later, Grandma who had recovered fully, badly injured her leg and her jaw after falling in the bathroom at home. She was unable to speak but was in stable condition, when admitted to a different hospital. She was supposed to have gone on vacation so we hadn't expected to hear from her and had no idea she was in the hospital. A few days later she began spiraling into critical condition. By the time the hospital called us, she was in the ICU, unconscious and critical. While I was on one phone trying to get a flight, my mom was on the other phone with the doctor who happened to be standing right outside Grandma's room. She begged him and then the nursing staff, to get a phone into her, so she could talk to her, for what looked like it would be the last time.

But at this hospital, the doctor and the nurses refused. While the doctor was on the phone with mom, Grandma, who had been unconscious just a few minutes before, unexpectedly opened her eyes and began to look around. The doctor told Mom what happened and took this as a sign that she her condition was turning around. Even so, Mom still pleaded with him to get a phone to Grandma. He told her there was no way to get a phone to an ICU patient. "We'll try and figure something out in the morning," he said, hanging up the phone. But Grandma didn't have until morning. She died just a few hours later, before we could get to her and we lost our chance to tell her we loved her – our chance to say goodbye.

Looking back on that time reminds me of that scripture, "without a vision, the people perish". Some people, even while facing serious illness or death are so self-motivated that just the possibility of dying makes them muster every ounce of strength they have, to fight it. But most people aren't like that. Most people need to use the strength of others – the people they love – to provide the strength they cannot find.

Patients need connection. They need vision – the vision to "see" themselves getting through the darkness and fear. They need help "seeing" the next day or the next week. Seeing themselves strong and well again. And without that strength and that support they so desperately need from the people they love, there is no vision. And without that vision, they perish.

Simply put, at that moment, Grandma needed us. That night, she needed to hear our voices and the very people who were there to be her advocates and to help her make that connection happen, didn't. And that night, Grandma perished, without knowing that we were on our way.

The good news is, the same thing that happened to us, doesn't have to happen at your facility. With just a few simple steps designed to help communication-impaired patients, you can not only make a huge difference in their lives, you might even save them.

Assessing Your Patient's Ability To Communicate

The next time you're caring for a patient with compromised communication ability, take a moment to see your patient's surroundings from her perspective. If your patient's family and friends can't be at the hospital with her, are there tools you can provide that will facilitate communication with the outside world?

Mobility Limitations

• If your patient can speak, is the telephone close enough to her for her to use?

• Does she need help dialing? Is she able to see well enough to read a phone number out of her address book or see the contacts on her smartphone?

• If your patient is unable to hold a telephone, would she benefit from a speakerphone or a cell phone?

Hearing/Speech Limitations

If your patient can't speak, ask her to indicate if she would like to have someone called for her, and task a patient representative or volunteer to hold the phone up to her ear and facilitate their communication.

If your patient is deaf, make sure that your facility has TTY telephones to connect with family members. If your patient is blind, make sure that she has Braille writers or other devices to help her communicate.

• Take a moment to call the department in your facility that deals with hearing or vision-impaired patients. They may have more tools or ideas that can bridge difficulties and enhance communication.

• Another idea for patients who can't speak, is patient Internet access. It can be a real lifesaver, allowing a patient to type an email, a text message or to supervise while a message is typed for them. If your facility doesn't have Internet access for patients, either you or another team member can use a smartphone to send an email or text a message for them, facilitating emergency communication with a loved one.

• For patients who have a temporary physically impairment, like a broken jaw, encourage them to use patient Internet access or their cell phones (if allowed) to email, text and keep in touch with family or children who might not be able to visit in person.

If you work with seriously ill pediatric or adult patients who need to communicate updates about their patient to a whole team of family and friends, there is a wonderful service called Care Pages. It was created by a family with a seriously ill child and no time to constantly email everyone who wanted to know how the child was doing. Care Pages provides free web sites to families enabling them to post pictures and messages from or about the patient without the painstaking task of having to update well meaning loved ones one by one! It gives families a way to reach out to others while spending quality time with the person who matters most – the patient. You can find more information at www.carepages.com .

Critical Care/End of Life

Since some hospitals don't provide patient Internet access in the ICU or CCU, you may have to get a bit more creative for patients in critical care units.

Fortunately technology has made huge strides in facilitating patient/family communication.

Even surgeons are now using Twitter to keep families apprised of patient's progress during surgery, while families who are apart during emergencies, are using Facebook and Twitter to keep each other up to date. You can use that same technology to help a critically ill or dying patient communicate with family members who might not make it to the hospital in time to be with them.

How? With a tablet or smartphone!

> "The next time you're caring for a patient with compromised communication ability, take a moment to look at her surroundings from her perspective."

Most tablets and smartphones have the ability to record video, audio and take photos, all of which can be sent or received via email right from the phone. Let's say you have a patient who might not make it through the night. His family is about to board a plane, but won't arrive for three or four hours. But if your unit has a tablet, the family can record a video or audio message and email it to you, so you can play it for the patient – something you can do without the Wi-Fi actually being on. Or they can email you a photo of themselves to show to the patient or an email that your patient can read for himself.

You can do the same thing at your end. Let's say that your patient is alert and oriented now, but you both realize that he might not live. Then you can use the tablet or phone to let him record a message to a loved one, that can later be emailed to the family. I don't think we have to tell anyone, how much that bit of video can mean to a family.

Or let's say that your patient is a John Doe or that she was a part of a mass casualty and even though you're relatively positive you have the right name with the right person, the family member is still in transit. You can snap a quick photo and email it to the family, hastening the identification.

Communication isn't just a patient's right – for many it can be their only link to the outside world, or a life-renewing source of strength and love. Combine that with outstanding medical care and watch the miracles flow. §

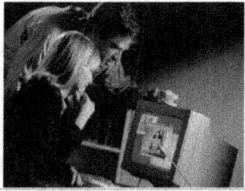

The Benefits of Patient Internet Access

According to Jennifer Lyons' chart, she's just a bad slip and fall who's lucky enough to be on her way to a full recovery. But to Jennifer, who is lying in bed with a broken mandible and broken limbs, nothing could be further from the truth. Jen was visiting the city on a business trip when her accident happened, and now she's lying in a bed 2,000 miles away from her family. Although her husband is flying in later tonight, never in her life has Jennifer felt more disconnected. That is, until her nurse points out the Internet monitor standing next to her bed. Even though she can't move her mouth, two minutes later, Jennifer is on Skype catching up with her children.

Two floors down, Rebecca Forrester is also lying in bed with no family members around her. She's in her eighties and the fall she took is already developing a complication – pneumonia. Her daughter is working in Tokyo and will take a day to get to her side – a day Rebecca may not have. With no telephones in this ICU, Rebecca knows if her daughter doesn't make it to her in time, she may never be able to speak to her again. Until a nurses' aide enters with a tablet. A minute later, Rebecca and her daughter are talking.

In a growing number of hospitals nationwide, hooking up your patients has just taken on a whole new meaning. Whether via tablets or bedside units, patient Internet access is revolutionizing patient care and patient communication.

Originally conceived as a way to reduce boredom and facilitate patient education, the units quickly began to add other features including relaxation videos, local TV channels, video games and telephones, besides videos and information patients can access on specific healthcare issues. The results show what medical professionals have suspected for years -- people simply feel better when they're active and connected with the world around them. But patient Internet manufacturers didn't stop there. They also found a way to add a host of applications that increase bedside patient care in ways never before possible, by bringing the information age right to the bedside.

But for the patients, it's all about facilitating communication whenever they need it – with loved ones, with friends or even with work. Just because someone is hospitalized doesn't mean they have to be isolated. For Jennifer Lyons, being able to communicate with her children means everything. Not only does she feel connected, because she can check in with them a few times a day, she feels more able to relax knowing that everything is fine at home.

As for Rebecca, she didn't fare as well. The pneumonia took hold and her daughter was unable to get to the hospital quickly enough to be with her before she passed away. But with the tablet and a little help from her nurses' aide, Rebecca and her daughter spent the rest of the day writing back and forth, telling stories, sharing memories and making sure they said everything to each other, that they wanted to say.

And to them, that made all the difference. Priceless.

The Tools

WORKING WITH ALZHEIMER'S PATIENTS

Are you dealing with an Alzheimer's patient? What is the best way to get the info from them that you need?

BY ELIZABETH HECK, MSW.

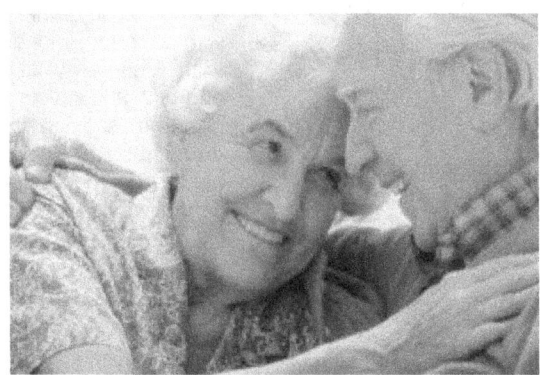

When you encounter an older adult in an emergency situation who appears confused and disoriented, the explanation may be Alzheimer's disease or a related dementia.

So how do you know you're dealing with an Alzheimer's patient? Clues can include withdrawal, lack of awareness or appreciation for the situation, blank, frightened or inappropriate facial expressions, or inability to track the passage of time.

A calm, confident, reassuring approach with the patient where you demonstrate to the person that you are in control of the situation is essential.

Speak slowly and clearly, using short sentences. Ask if the person wears any assistive devices such as glasses or hearing aids and help to locate them.

Be aware of the surroundings -- a hectic environment can be over stimulating and may lead to a catastrophic reaction. Try to talk to the person in a quiet room or area away from excess activity. Cognitive impairment may affect medical decision making ability.

When it is determined that a person lacks decision making capacity, identifying a surrogate can be a challenge.

You may not always be looking for a traditional next of kin but rather a close friend, live in companion, neighbor or public guardian. Sources for identifying surrogate decision makers include advance directives, medic alert bracelet, **the Safe Return bracelet** (see below), or an ID card in person's wallet that states the memory impairment. The person with Alzheimer's disease may not be able to provide reliable information and may even mention the name of a deceased relative or loved one. It is best to identify or confirm information through other documentation or other sources.

Keep in mind that persons with a mild cognitive impairment may still have decision-making capacity for some choices regarding medical treatment.

QUICK TIPS

SAFE RETURN

Safe Return is a national, government-funded program of the Alzheimer Association that assists in the identification and safe, timely return of individuals with Alzheimer's disease and related dementias who wander off, sometimes far from home, and become lost. The Alzheimer's Association Safe Return Program is the only nationwide program of its kind. Since the program began in 1993, over 115,000 individuals have registered in Safe Return nationwide. The program has facilitated the recovery of more than 9,000 individuals to their families and caregivers with an over 99% success in safely returning those registered in the program.

For more information about The Alzheimer's Association Safe Return Program or to register someone please visit www.alz.org/safereturn or call 888-572-8566. Assistance is available 24 hours a day, seven days a week.

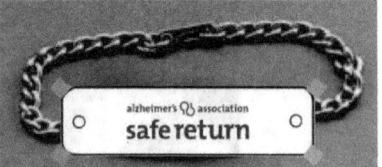

Even if the person cannot comprehend complex situations, they may still be able to make simple decisions or provide an opinion regarding treatment.

According to a recently released study (Hebert et al, 2003) on prevalence in the United States, an estimated 4.5 million Americans have Alzheimer's disease. With the aging of the population and the baby boom generation, data shows that by 2050, the number of Americans with Alzheimer's could range from 11.3 million to 16 million. More than 7 out of 10 people with Alzheimer's disease live at home and most of the care is provided by family and friends.

Unlike other medical disorders, Alzheimer's disease is not easily recognized. Health care providers need to be informed about the signs, symptoms and situations common to persons with Alzheimer's disease.

Here are a few examples of situations that might result in a trip to the ED for people with Alzheimer's disease.

Wandering – Over 60% of persons with a diagnosis of Alzheimer's disease will wander or become lost. Individuals can become lost and disoriented even in familiar surroundings.

Falls – According to the C.D.C. (2002), falls are the leading cause of injury deaths among older adults. Falls can occur when a person is wandering, attempts to get out of a wheelchair or get over bedside rails.

Appearance of intoxication – Some of the symptoms of Alzheimer's could cause the mistaken impression that the person is intoxicated, such as visual deficits, language impairment, personality changes, and irritability.

Traffic violations/auto accidents – A person with Alzheimer's disease may speed, slow down, not respond to traffic signals or become lost while driving.

ISABEL

ONE FAMILY'S AWARD WINNING SOLUTION TO THE PROPER DIAGNOSIS AND TREATMENT OF COMPLICATED ILLNESSES

After a simple bout with the chicken pox developed into nearly fatal complications, multiple organ failure and cardiac arrest, three year old Isabel Maude spent two months in the hospital – including a month in Intensive Care.

All this, because her family doctor and local emergency department failed to recognize that the symptoms she was developing were known chicken pox complications. Isabel was finally diagnosed with Toxic Shock Syndrome and Necrotizing Fasciitis. Luckily Isabel escaped with her life and without brain damage, but the close call didn't escape her physician or her parents.

Jason and Charlotte Maude partnered with Dr. Joseph Britto M.D., in 1999 to create Isabel, is an award-winning, clinical decision support system, named after the child who inspired it.

Its unique feature is a diagnosis reminder system which instantly provides the clinician a checklist of likely diagnoses in the clinical workflow.

By finding specific answers to clinical questions arising in the workflow, Isabel serves as a single entry point to search medical knowledge. Isabel uses unique concept matching techniques as opposed to standard key word searches.

Dr Joseph Britto conceived the structure of the system, that can help improve the quality of care in hospital and family practice, either as a stand alone web based system or embedded in an electronic medical record.

Within months of its launch, the system attracted over 20,000 users from over 100 countries. Impressed with the system's high levels of speed and accuracy, demand rapidly grew for an adult version. This is currently underway and will be launched in late 2004. Initially funded by The Isabel Medical Charity (a UK registered charity), the Isabel product range is now delivered by the charity's fully owned commercial subsidiary, Isabel Healthcare Ltd. . §

For sales information contact ussales@isabelhealthcare.com

http://www.isabelhealthcare.com

Isabel Healthcare Ltd.
PO Box 28832 LONDON SW13 9DZ
UK **TEL**. +44 (0)208 748 4330

They may also be the cause or the victim of an auto accident.

Elder Abuse/Self Neglect – A person may live alone, yet no longer be able to provide for their basic needs.

Or they might have a caregiver who is not able to provide for their needs or who is abusing them. Warning signs to look for include a disheveled appearance, poor hygiene, poor nutrition or hydration, inability to

manage medication, bruises, welts, frequent use of hospitals or doctors, soiled clothing or bedding, or the lack of necessities or personal effects.

Correctly identifying a patient as having Alzheimer's will help you provide the best care possible for your patient while allowing you to get his family or surrogate decision maker on the scene as soon as possible. §

MANAGING MASS CASUALTY SITUATIONS

How to do it right way from the doctor who wrote the book on triage – on September 11th

BY DR. SUSAN BRIGGS, MD. FACS

Disasters follow no rules. No one can predict the location, time, or complexity of the next disaster, be it natural, man-made and terrorism.

For local hospitals, after dealing with the initial triage, the largest impact on emergency departments is that large numbers of casualties make victim identification difficult due to the physical and/or psychological injuries sustained by victims of an unexpected disaster. This causes significant stress to victims, victims' families and to medical providers. As physicians and nurses, our first reaction is to provide our patients with the best care with their immediate needs and medical background in mind. But unsettling as it is, when we're triaging critically injured, unconscious patients we've never seen before, and no next to nothing about, the best-case scenario takes a back seat.

As the Supervising Medical Officer of the National Disaster Medical Assistance Team (DMAT), no one knows that feeling better than Dr. Susan Briggs. Dr. Briggs, called to head up triage efforts at Ground Zero on September 11th, is no stranger to disaster management, having headed up triage and medical efforts at the site of many major events including earthquakes and hurricanes.

From her experience Dr. Briggs has learned that organization is the key to keeping chaos at a minimum. The condition of arriving patients, usually hinges on the type of mass casualty alert.

For a local emergency, like recent nightclub fires or large multi-car pileups, patients will probably be brought directly to the hospital, with basic treatment occurring only by paramedics or fire personnel. In the case of a large-scale alert, like 9/11 with DMAT's on scene, most of the critically injured will already have been seen, received initial triage assessment and treatment and been directed to the right facility. Then there are major mass casualty alerts where the hospital and its personnel may be physically impacted as well, as in the case of an earthquake.

The first line of defense for any type of mass casualty alert, is a clear, easy to use emergency plan with frequent drills, so personnel will know precisely what to do when disaster strikes. In mass casualty situations like 9/11, victims will be taken to casualty stabilization sites and then transferred to multiple medical facilities, depending on the number, severity and type of casualties.

Here are a few simple things you can add to your usual emergency department procedures, that will help your team hasten the identification and notification process from the moment victims come through the door.

1) Add a few lines to the emergency intake sheet that you normally use for mass casualty situations, to include the location that the victim was found, a place for the paramedics or the person who brought him in, to jot down any other information he has on the patient, and a quick description of any personal effects brought in with him. This can help match patients to their belongings and contact information later on, or help their families identify them by the approximate location in which they were found.

2) For facilities with emergency patient tracking software or EMR, ask your software vendor if your software can be adapted to add a section to capture the above information. According to St. Vincent's ED, the Level One trauma center closest to the World Trade Center, adding new field choices under "mode of arrival" to include types of arrival (i.e., rescue worker or civilian rescuer, as well as choices that allowed them to track if a patient was victim of the tragedy, a rescue worker or a non-disaster related patient), enabled them to quickly determine their current patient population at the touch of a button. For overwhelmed ED staffers and families trying to find their loved ones, this type of system flexibility is invaluable.

3) During a major mass casualty situation, keep in mind that a clearing house may need to be established, to facilitate calls from frantic family members looking for information on their loved ones.

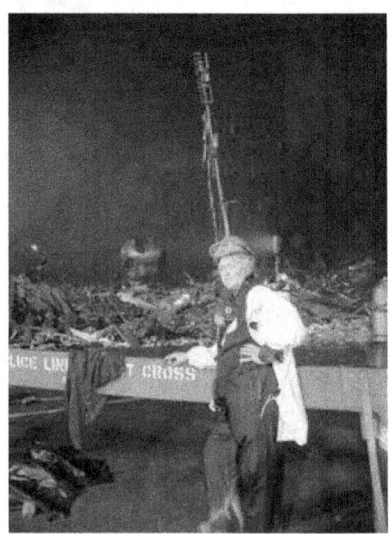

Dr. Susan Briggs at Ground Zero

If a hotline hasn't been established a few hours after the event, work with police, fire and the media to set up a hotline that victim's families can call regarding information. For the hospital's part, you'll need to assign one or two staff members from your media relations department to work with emergency personnel, as a touch point for information that needs to be funneled to local radio and TV stations. This way they can broadcast the central number for families to call regarding information or a central location for families to report missing individuals.   Depending on the type of emergency and the size of your facility, your hospital should also be prepared to act as that central location. It's also a good idea to have the media urge the public not to attempt to call or visit local hospitals, until they have spoken to the hotline or confirmed that their family member is in a specific facility.

4) Organization may be the most important part of successful emergency management, but flexibility is a close second.

On 9/11, Dr. Briggs, assembled her team of DMATs, and briefed them on their initial mission, to set up a full service major and minor emergency room to treat and triage survivors, just a few moments away from Ground Zero. She left them to their work and attended the first briefing, where she was told that very few people trapped in the twin towers had survived. Moments later, she returned with the most current information, and their initial tent set-up quickly changed to a four-quadrant medical services area -- respiratory care, acute wound care,   orthopedic care, and advanced cardiac life support -- along with an advanced trauma-life support area, with full defibrillation and resuscitation capabilities, to care mainly for rescue workers.

> "Organization may be the most important part of successful mass casualty alert management, but (maintaining) flexibility is a close second."

The team also found out that the majority of those who had survived had sustained third degree burns.

This enabled them to mobilize their team of burn specialists to the Cornell Burn Unit to help Cornell's team handle those patients.

Had the DMATs not been able to accurately assess the situation as it unfolded, and been flexible enough to shift their capabilities to meet the needs of the event, life saving treatment would have been seriously delayed.

To prepare for such an emergency, every hospital that doesn't have a major mass casualty team already on call, should put together a database of their staffer's specialties, such as special clinical skills dealing with crush injuries and limb reattachment, full thickness burns or pediatric trauma, as well as any other skills that might be crucial, like the languages the speak or special administrative or training dealing with the media.

5) Dealing with people with special needs. During a disaster, special needs persons without injuries are of significant concern due to their chronic medical needs and will often be placed in a "special needs" shelter to ensure the best medical care. Your facility should be aware of the patient population of your area, in order to provide care or services to the elderly or special needs patients as the need arises, during a major mass casualty.

During 9/11 and the 2003 Manhattan blackout, police and fire personnel went door to door in the affected areas to make sure that the elderly, infirm, or those with respiratory difficulties were out of the danger zone and had the medical equipment and supplies that they needed to stay well. It's a good idea to have a basic plan in place to help serve your community's special needs.

6) Lastly, in the case of a major disaster, like an earthquake or large-scale event, make sure that you and your staffers have everything you need to take care of yourselves. For example in California, hospitals have large sealed trash cans filled with enough supplies, including water, flashlights, canned food etc, to supply each staffer with everything they would need to survive for two or three days in the event of an earthquake or other emergency. Since most hospitals have plenty of first aid supplies and food supplies, they don't always think of putting together disaster supplies for staff members. But as we all know, in a disaster anything can happen. Food sources like cafeterias can be leveled or inaccessible. Or what looks like a huge supply of first aid equipment, flashlights and batteries can quickly dwindle. Your staff can only help others if they have the food, water and supplies that they need to keep themselves healthy. So make sure you draft and review worst case scenarios with your team, to make sure you're as prepared as possible for any eventuality. §

PEDIATRIC NOTIFICATIONS

If you thought handling next of kin notification for adults was tough, try critically ill children

BY CATHLEEN SHANAHAN, RN, BSN, MS, CMTE

If you think handling notifications for your adult patients is tough, try critically ill children. For me, as the head of the trauma department at one of America's top pediatric facilities, Chicago's Lurie Children's Hospital, having to notifying parents that their children have been the victims of trauma or identify pediatric Jane Does, is an every day occurrence. But just because we look like we're handling it well, doesn't mean that it ever becomes routine.

When a child comes into our ED without a parent, it's usually the result of an accident or traumatic event. Even though our first priority is to tend to the child's medical needs, our next priority is to identify the child. We need to get his parents or guardian down to the hospital, to give consent for his treatment, provide vital medical history and most importantly, to be at their child's side when he needs them most.

You'd be surprised how often a child is brought into Lurie Children's without anything pointing to his or her identity. Many times it's the result of a car accident, where the parents are injured as well as the child, and are taken to another hospital, while the child is brought here for specialized pediatric treatment. Since children don't have driver's licenses or checkbooks, identifying a child can be challenging.

Just the other day, three children ranging from 8 months to 3 years were brought into our ED after a serious automobile accident.

Their parents, who were in bad shape, were taken to another hospital and the paramedics had no clue about their names, ages or medical history. We began their medical evaluation and as we always do when dealing with an unidentified child, opening a trauma pack for each, using a patient number to identify them. We estimated their ages, did a full physical description including any identifying marks and clothing, then ordered a full set of x-rays, which helps to identify any conditions or injuries that aren't readily apparent.

Our biggest asset in this situation was the solid relationships that we've built with police, fire department, and other local hospitals – as we work together to get the children identified as quickly as possible. After a major accident like this, the police and fire department were already in the ED coordinating efforts. With our special emergency landline system we're instantly linked by phone with any local hospital we need to reach. As my team began calling to find out where the children's parents were taken, hospitals began to call us, to say, "I know you're looking for the mom and dad of the accident victims. They're not here," saving us precious time. In this case, we found the hospital relatively quickly and found out that even though the children's parents had been seriously injured, the children's caregiver who had also been in the accident, was fine. The hospital sent her over to Lurie Children's and she – and later on the parents – were able to give us all the information we needed to identify and treat the children.

In the case of a completely unidentified child, especially babies, we depend on our procedures. Usually the fire department, police or DCFS dropped the child off, so they are already aware of the situation and have already begun going through the child's clothing and personal effects to gather evidence and identify the child. We'll send the police or paramedics right back to the scene to gather additional information, medicine bottles, names, and to canvass the area. There is almost always someone who saw something. Someone from pastoral care automatically comes down and a social worker will get involved if it looks like any abuse was involved.

QUICK TIPS

THE NATIONAL NEXT OF KIN REGISTRY

The National Next Of Kin Registry was created to expedite and assist State and Local Agencies in locating and notifying the Next Of Kin of a deceased family member. The passing of a loved one is a difficult transition for family and friends. This sad time is compounded when you're not informed when a loved one passes on. This happens often when State and Local Agencies are unable to locate a family member or next of kin. The content of this web site focuses on locating family of the deceased. This registry can also be used to locate kin for those who have been critically injured or those with Alzheimer's. To request an emergency search, contact a local Law Enforcement Agency. For more information, contact Mark Cerney Project Manager, National Next Of Kin Registry www.nokr.org

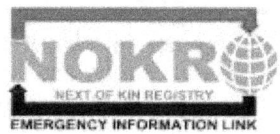

Together, they take care of figuring out where we go from here, while our team takes care of the child medically.

If these steps don't elicit any clues to the child's identity, we'll get media affairs involved. We will never show the face or reveal the name of any child. Instead, we photograph the child's clothing and personal effects and release it to the media along with the child's estimated age, description and the vicinity in which she was found. We work closely with detectives and DCFS to give them all the details they need to chase down any leads they get from the public. Many times just calling DCFS or the police will locate parents or bring about an identification. In the case of severe trauma, abuse or inflicted injury, we always balance treating the child, with carefully gathering as much evidence as possible, to help the eventual police investigation. We had a young girl a few years ago, whose brutal attacker was convicted mainly on the evidence gathered and catalogued in the trauma room.

When it comes to providing emergency contact information, kids aren't always the best source. We have seven or eight year old kids come in everyday, who I'm sure are sophisticated in every other way. But get them in a trauma situation and ask them what their mom's name is and they'll say it's "mom". In this case, the first thing we'll do is look at whatever they brought in with them. School-age kids almost always have a backpack. If we don't find anything there, we'll check our records to see if the child is in our system and begin to gently probe the child for information. We ask them where their house is, what their school looks like, information about their friend's houses, maybe a familiar landmark on the corner like a 7/11 or the name of a park. If you can't find their contact information right away, try to find the name of their school. Their books will probably have the name

> "We have seven or eight year old kids come in everyday, who I'm sure are sophisticated in every other way. But get them in a trauma situation and ask them what their mom's name is and they'll say it's 'mom'."

of their school stamped inside.

Schools are also a great source for emergency contact information. They'll often even list alternate people to call in an emergency if the parents are at work or hard to reach. In an emergency, schools will usually send someone directly down to the hospital with the child's emergency card and emergency consent forms. If the injury occurs at school, most schools will send someone from the school along with the child to the hospital, while someone else is calling the parent. As a parent myself, I would suggest that every parent name someone else on the child's emergency card, who knows the child well and would be able to step in to help out during an emergency if the parents can't get there right away.

So once you identify a child, how do you know if the person who comes to the hospital is really his parent or relative? It's not always easy. Remember that the parents didn't expect to have to come to the hospital today, and probably won't be carrying three forms of ID and their child's birth certificate. For people that come in and say they're related to a child who's been in the media, we get as much ID as we can, be it a driver's license, pictures or other proof. With kids, the biggest test is to watch their response when that person goes in the room. Usually you'll here a resounding "Mom!" or "Daddy!" and you know you've got the right person. If there's no response from the kid, or if they're not sure of the adult, it's probably not the right person. Or worse, the child might recoil from the adult which could

indicate an abusive situation.

Treating kids also means caring for their parents. When I have to make a notification call I'll begin by telling the person on the phone who I am and ask them how they are related to the child. If it's the mom or dad, I'll tell them that their child has been brought to Lurie Children's Hospital. Of course the parent will immediately ask how the child is. This is always the hardest part of the call. If the child is clearly fine, I'll say "Don't worry, they're fine, we just need you to come down here." But if there is a more serious injury, or if the child hasn't survived, I tell them that the child has been in an accident, that they need to come down, and if necessary, that we need to get their medical history. If they refuse to get off the phone until they find out what's wrong, I'll say that we're very concerned about their child's health and that they need to come down right away. I always try to calm the person down as much as I can – tell them to go and get a pencil and paper to take down the address of the hospital, to take down my name and my number. I tell them to ask for me right away when they get here so they don't have to waste any time at the desk and then try to make sure they have someone to drive them over. I also remind them that they need to drive carefully and slowly and to make sure that they get there in one piece! At Lurie Children's our top priority is the restoration of the health of every child who comes through our door, no matter who they are and where they come from. §

NOT YOUR "RUN OF THE MILL" NOTIFICATIONS

What to do when your patient is a John Doe, homeless, or doesn't speak English

BY RICHARD FANTUS, MD, FACS, ELIZABETH HECK, MSW & DORATHY PEREZ, RN, BSN

Nobody looks in the mirror in the morning and says to himself, I am going to get into a car accident today! But it's exactly that ephemeral nature of emergencies that makes trauma such a challenge to even the best organized, most talented health care team.

Traumatic injuries produce just that – trauma – not only from a medical standpoint, but from a personal standpoint. The patient on that gurney, in pain and totally helpless, deserves the best care possible. And that means, care given with his specific needs in mind. That's fine when you've known and treated this patient for years and are holding his full set of medical records. Not an easy task when you're seeing this critically injured patient for the first time and don't have a clue about his medical history.

Traumatic injuries create situations where patient information may be totally absent – including something as basic as your patient's name.

Without a conscious patient to verbally provide this information, it's necessary to look through whatever personal information the patient may have with him. From scraps of paper to video store rental cards, we try to piece together the story of his life. All this, while the clock is races against us.

But what happens, after all your searching, if your patient is a John Doe? Since our medical center is in one of the busiest metropolitan centers possible, time is always of the essence. So we make sure preparations are made prior to the patient's arrival. One of the ways we do it, is to prepare a chart as a Jane or John Doe and assign it a unique identifier. The patient will remain a John Doe in our patient tracking system until we are able to identify him.

And without an identity there can be no next of kin notification, or medical history. In order to address this crucial issue we put together a John Doe identification policy several years ago.

At our institution, as in many Level I trauma centers, we have a crisis worker as a member of our trauma team. Their role is to work to identify the John Doe, to determine next of kin and start the notification process.

There is an algorithm that is followed with several steps to attempt to identify a patient. These steps range from examining all of the patient's belongings for clues to his identity, to having the police department finger print the patient and search databases for matches of those who were fingerprinted for security clearance. §

WHEN THE ED'S EFFORTS TURN UP NO LEADS...

When the ED and trauma team's measures fail, the task of finding a patient's identity and next of kin falls to the Social Services department.

For Elizabeth Heck who spent many years in the trenches, being called in to save the day, became second nature. In many cases she has the hospital's PR department enlist the media to appeal to their viewing audience.

Careful to follow HIPAA protocol for patient privacy, the PR department has shown pictures of the patient's personal effects or has given out particulars of the event and asked for the public's help in reporting anything that they might have witnessed.

One of her most unusual cases concerned a man who was discovered just outside of the hospital entrance doors. He kept saying over and over, "I just want to go home. Somebody help me, please."

The man appeared confused and disoriented. He was an African American gentleman who seemed to be in his eighties. Even though he was unshaven and disheveled, his clothes appeared fairly new and tailored, and his hair neatly trimmed. He didn't strike us as just another homeless person peddling near the hospital doors. There was definitely something not quite right with the situation. He had urinated all over himself, stated he was thirsty and was complaining of chest pain. He needed medical attention.

One of the nurses escorted him to the Emergency Department, explaining that he was discovered just outside of the hospital. After finding no identification on him, they began a John Doe chart and a physician assessed and treated his medical needs. One of the ED staff members gave him some water and a sandwich, helped him get into some clean clothes and began to ask him some questions. He said his name was Ray and that he lived with his wife in San Francisco. Although the information he provided was pretty sketchy, it appeared that this man could have wandered away from home and had been unable to retrace his steps.

The staff contacted the San Francisco Police but they couldn't find a report of a missing person from that area.

Since the case required more investigation and a possible transfer to a local county hospital, the social worker was called in. She contacted the police department again and suggested that they contact all of the area police departments for a missing person report, providing them an accurate description of the John Doe. As it turned out, another police department in a suburb outside of San Francisco, did have a missing person report meeting his description. A photo that the wife of our John Doe had provided to the police, was scanned and sent to us electronically. Bingo! We had a match.

Ray, was born and grew up in San Francisco, but now lived in the suburb with his wife. Because of clinical dementia, he lived more in the past than the present and home to him, will always be San Francisco. When his caregiver was making lunch, he decided he'd like a haircut. Not liking the caregiver's reply that they would have to wait until the next day to go out, he slipped out the door and got on a bus, becoming hopelessly lost. Thanks to the police and some quick thinking by the social worker, Ray made it back home to his family, safe and sound. §

WHEN YOUR JOHN DOE IS HOMELESS

The patient, known only as John Doe, was difficult to see under the hodgepodge of tubing, the quiet clicking of the ventilator the room's only sound.

From all appearances he was homeless, but in the opinion of his nurse, who has had vast experience in dealing with patients just like him, everyone has a mother or a father, a son or a daughter, and homeless or not, it's a nurse's responsibility to do what he can to help find them. Usually it's just a matter of taking that extra

> "Homeless people are very savvy and self-sufficient... They write important phone numbers on the insides of a hat, put them in their shoes, or sew numbers inside the seams of their coat..."

few minutes to connect the dots.

"Homeless people are very savvy and self-sufficient when it comes to survival skills," he explains. "They write important phone numbers on the insides of a hat, put them in their shoes, or sew numbers inside the seams of their coats. I go through every stitch of clothing."

If that doesn't turn up any emergency contact numbers or personal information, he examines the patient's body for needle tracks, scars or tattoos and if necessary, sends fingerprints to the police for a background check.

Sometimes the police's theory is that the homeless person had a desire to be a loner, and they see no need to reconnect them with their family after they are injured or dead. But the nurse is quick to disagree.

"Things change, [and] these people are still human beings. I believe that every homeless person is still a father or mother, [or a] son or daughter to somebody out there. These people may have done things they are not proud of, they may have mental illness, but their family has a right to know what happened to them."

From a hospital's perspective, a patient without an identity is a patient without funding. But once a nurse or a social worker positively IDs a patient as a US citizen, the hospital can help the patient apply for Medicaid and then get reimbursement for the bill.

"Identifying people is a reasonable endeavor. It is part of a holistic approach. When you locate family, you find a surrogate to speak on behalf of the patient, to be an advocate.

The family should decide on the patient's follow-up and if the patient has died, the family should decide where they are buried." §

DEALING WITH NON-ENGLISH SPEAKING PATIENTS

For Emergency Departments, dealing with patients for whom English is not a first language, can be difficult. But when that problem is compounded by a patient who is unconscious, or unable to communicate her medical history, it makes the situation even more difficult.

Tenet Healthcare has approached that situation proactively, by making the decision to provide comprehensive care to every community its facilities touch. During recruiting, they take into consideration the communities the facility serves, and choose staffers who are from the country or culture that they need. When dealing with patients and their families, being able to speak a language from taking a few courses doesn't always cut it. Tenet wants people who are culturally able to deal with their patients, to give them the care and respect they deserve with their particular needs in mind.

One Tenet hospital has staffers who speak twenty-two different languages! Each of their hospitals maintains a database of workers who speak languages other than English, along with the shift they work, so when the need arises for an interpreter, they can immediately call the appropriate person to communication with the patient and her family. §

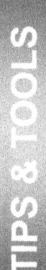

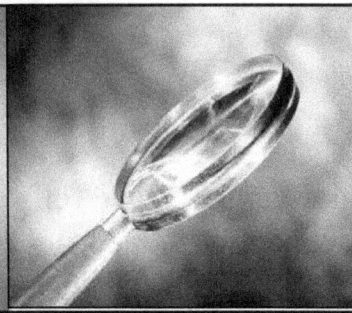

Quick Tips For Finding Contact Information

Where To Look For Patient's Emergency Contact Information

- Inside their Wallet
- Driver's License
- Credit Cards
- Photo /Company ID Card
- Smartphone, Phone Contacts, Speed Dial
- Information on flash drives, CDs
- Medic Alert or Safe Return Bracelet

- ICE Contact
- Personal Address book
- Insurance Card
- Business Cards
- Contacts on their Notebook Computer or Tablet
- Email addresses or Web Sites

- Name on the Letterhead of any Business Correspondence
- Contact Page of their Date Book
- In the Glove Compartment or on the Visor of their Car
- Their Car Registration or License Plate
- Inside Shoewallet

Advice From Ground Zero 9/11

"To prepare for Mass Casualty Incidents, add a few lines to your emergency intake sheet, to include the location that the victim was found, a place for the paramedics or person who brought him in, to jot down any other information on the patient, and a quick description of any personal effects brought in with him. This can help match patients to their belongings and contact information later on, or help their families identify them using the approximate location in which they were found."

Where To Look For Children's Emergency Contact Information

- Book Bags and Lunch Boxes
- School Name Stamped in School Books
- Names in Notebooks on Homework, Work Sheets
- ICE Contact, Smartphone Speed Dial or Contacts

- Medic Alert Bracelet
- iPod Touch Contacts or Inside Phone/iPod Case
- Inside Their Clothes or Underwear
- Names & Numbers of Friends
- Previous Hospital Records or Birth Records

Advice From Lurie Children's Hospital/Chicago

"School-age kids almost always have a backpack. If we don't find anything there, we'll check our records to see if the child is in our system and begin to gently probe the child for information. We ask them where their house is, what their school looks like, information about their friend's houses, maybe a familiar landmark on the corner like a 7/11 or the name of a park..."

Dealing with John Does Amnesia & Dementia Patients

Look for key ring/convenience cards from grocery or video rental stores. If you find a convenience card on your patient's key ring and can't identify the patient in any other way, call the store, tell them you have an emergency and have them give you or contact the patient's home number.

Check to see if the patient has a Safe Return Bracelet from the Alzheimer's Association or a piece of Medic-Alert jewelry. If they do, contact the toll free number to locate emergency contact information.

If you only have a patient's address but no phone number, or a location where an incident took place, try looking it up in the Haines Criss + Cross Directory, or other reverse directory. To get a copy of the directory, go to their web site at http://www.criss-cross.com/ or call 800-254-3449.

Even if your patient has amnesia, if he is able to talk, be sure to listen carefully to everything he says. People may remember a name or a place. One patient began repeating numbers apparently at random. A nurse began to write it down and realized it could be parts of a phone number. When they called it, they reached his grandmother in Canada. Another time emergency personnel found a man's identity because he was able to remember the name of a store. They called it and found out that a friend there had been desperately searching for him.

If the patient appears to be homeless, look at all of his clothing, even in the seams of his shirt, inside his hat or for papers sewn into the lining of their coat. Many homeless people have been known to safeguard this information in case of emergency.

If the patient is unconscious or has no identification anywhere on his body, the trauma team will need to get a complete description of the patient, noting all identifying marks and any details of the location where he was found, then notify the local police to check to see if he's been reported missing. Fingerprinting may also aid in identification.

If all else fails, try showing photos of the patient's personal effects, as well as circumstances surrounding the incident or accident, in the media. Be sure to hold a few details back, so that you can be sure the person calling is actually a relative of the patient. Have the description of the patient sent to the front desk personnel and ED staff as well. If a person comes to the hospital searching for a patient whose name isn't found on the patient roster, ask for a description of the person they're seeking – it just may be your John Doe. When a match seems to be imminent, have that family member or friend present evidence that they are indeed related to, or a friend of the patient, and note all of the proceedings in the patient's medical record.

Google It!

"If you find a name or an email address or even a company name on your patient, and have no other clues to go on, don't forget to Google it. Typing the small facts you know into a search engine can fill in the details. A person's name plus a company name can give you their contact number, a link to Facebook. Twitter, LinkedIn or web site. And from there, you can easily find their friends or contact information."

FAMILY IN THE ER

Re-examining the practice of limiting access for patient families during emergency procedures

Based on a study by DORRIE FONTAINE, RN, DNSc, FAAN & **KATHY ROBINSON,** RN

Despite growing support for allowing family members to be present during emergency medical procedures, only five of U.S. hospitals have written policies permitting such access during CPR or invasive procedures, according to a new survey of nurses co-sponsored by the Emergency Nurses Association (ENA) and the American Association of Critical-Care Nurses (AACN) and published jointly in the *Journal of Emergency Nursing* ™ and the *American Journal of Critical Care*®.

In addition, approximately one-quarter of responding nurses say family presence is still prohibited for both resuscitation and invasive procedures, despite guidelines to the contrary.

"When patients are in literally a life-or-death situation, their loved ones should be with them whenever possible," said one of the study's co-authors, Dorrie Fontaine, RN, DNSc, FAAN, president-elect of AACN and associate dean for academic programs at the University of California at San Francisco (UCSF) School of Nursing. "Having family present during emergency procedures can be a great source of comfort and support for patients." Such situations typically occur in adult and newborn intensive care units and in emergency departments.

"A decade of research shows that the presence of family members during invasive emergency procedures can be helpful to families, healthcare providers and the patients themselves," added Kathy Robinson, RN, president of ENA and EMS

Program Manager for the Pennsylvania Department of Health. "Yet despite growing support for family presence during emergency procedures, too many physicians and other healthcare practitioners resist adopting this practice."

The survey was sent to members of American Association of Critical-Care Nurses and the Emergency Nurses Association. Among its findings, reported in the May 2003 edition of the *American Journal of Critical Care* and the upcoming June 2003 issue of the *Journal of Emergency Nursing*:

•About one-quarter of nurses reported that family presence was prohibited for CPR (29 percent) and invasive procedures (25 percent), even though their units had no written policies prohibiting such access.

•Only five percent of respondents worked in units that had written policies allowing such access.

•Family members ask to be present for such procedures approximately one-third to two-thirds of the time (31 percent for resuscitation, 61 percent for invasive procedures).

On the more positive side, approximately half of all units covered by the survey allow family presence without a written policy (45 percent for resuscitation and 51 percent for invasive procedures).

"The option should exist in all hospitals backed up by a written policy," Fontaine said. "There also should be education so staff members can effectively support families in deciding whether to be present during emergency procedures or resuscitation. An ongoing follow-up mechanism should evaluate the effectiveness of the policy and ensure

that the rights of patients and their families are always respected."

Robinson agreed, saying, "Many ED managers and hospital administrators may not be aware of the research that has been done on family presence. Also, many may not know how to use the findings to develop guidelines and policies, customize a staff education program, or how to successfully facilitate family presence practices. Families are much more resilient under these circumstances than many health care providers think. Anticipated problems during resuscitation in hospitals that adopt this practice have not materialized and in fact, most times it helps families realize that everything possible was done' to save their loved ones."

Previous studies have found multiple benefits for family presence during medical emergencies, including:

•Removing doubts about what is happening to the patient;

•Reducing anxiety and fear;

•Providing feelings of support and help to the patient;

•Sustaining patient-family connectedness;

•Facilitating the grief process, and

•Engendering feelings of being helpful to the healthcare staff.

Fontaine and Robinson agreed that the nation's critical care and emergency department nurses, who are the most continually and intimately involved with seriously ill patients and their families, should work closely with physicians and healthcare administrators to adopt more widespread policies supporting family access during emergency procedures.

"It is the responsibility, if not duty, of every nurse to make the option of family presence a key part of any hospital stay," Fontaine concluded. §

ED/Family Patient Assistants Let Nurses Focus on Patient Care

Finding a shelter for a homeless patient, tracking down the family of an automobile crash victim, and holding the hand of a nursing home transfer patient are not part of an emergency nurse's official job description, but they are all things that need to be done every day in emergency departments (EDs). Luckily, ED nurses at St. John's Hospital in Springfield, Missouri, have a staff resource to take care of patient and family needs that are not directly related to patient care.

As the only Level I adult/pediatric trauma center in the region, St. John's Hospital provides emergency care to 65,000 patients each year, including vacationers from nearby Branson, Missouri. A new emergency trauma center that will increase their bed capacity from 31 to 45 will open this summer.

"We want our nurses to take care of each patient like they would want their own family members treated if they were lying in that bed," stated Toni Hawkins, RN, clinical manager of the emergency trauma center. "But we all know the ED can be chaotic, and we don't always have time to provide the TLC component as much as we want to."

That is where the family/patient assistants (FPAs) come in. These staff members perform a variety of duties, including serving as informational liaisons between doctors and families; notifying families of a patient's status; finding transportation for patients; and calling on pastoral care services when needed. The ED has 24-hour FPA coverage.

"We make sure the patients and families are well aware of what's going on," explained Maxine Coggins, who has been an FPA at St. John's for 20 years. "The doctors will tell us, 'Tell (the patient) the tests are back, and I'll be in soon.' We go from room to room to make sure the patients are all aware of what they're waiting on. If someone is traveling through the area and is involved in an accident, a big part of our job is to find and notify the families."

Supporting the ED staff is another one of the FPA's main priorities. "We do try to support them in as many ways as possible," Coggins noted. "Many times the nurses are just too busy to spend that family time. Should we get a trauma in, they don't have time to stop and notify the family, so that's a major role for us." FPAs can spend hours searching for family members of motor vehicle accident victims by contacting the local highway patrol, or calling on area colleges to pull up student identification photos in the middle of the night. "I think it frees up the nurses and takes a tremendous burden off of them," Coggins said. "They don't have to worry about whether a family has been notified, and they know the family is not going to come bursting through the door."

Once a patient's family arrives, the FPA is responsible for keeping them informed. The FPA takes all incoming calls for ED patients on a cordless phone. "We have to be very careful of the information we give out - that's a big responsibility," Coggins noted.

The FPA position is also the family members' link to pastoral care. "If we have a code come in, we notify the chaplain, and we're there to meet the family when they arrive. If the patient doesn't survive, we work closely with the chaplain to meet the family's needs," Coggins said. "It's a very encompassing position, - we have to have just the right person with the right personality," Hawkins added. "They have to be able to talk to people easily, and be someone patients and families feel comfortable with." All FPAs go through a hospital and departmental preceptor program, and they receive a resource manual developed especially for their position. "We've actually had other hospitals come and model our program," she said.

"When I started this 21 years ago, they didn't necessarily want a person with a lot of training," recalled Coggins. They wanted someone they felt could be warm with families, could relate to the families - they called us the mothers to the ED, though we've kind of outgrown that now."

Coggins brings another special quality to her role as an FPA. Thirteen years ago she witnessed her son's accidental death when the dune buggy he was driving was hit by a car. Her decision to return to her position at St. John's after a period of mourning was inspired by a resolve to help other families through the devastating experience of losing a loved one. "My sole purpose is to let families know that you can survive," she said. "I had to decide whether to use my experience, and I decided to use it. Every time you take a step in your life, it just helps you relate to the patients and families." § For more information about St. John's Hospital's FPA program, contact Toni Hawkins at thawkins@sprg.smhs.com.

COULD A HOSPITAL FIND <u>YOUR</u> CONTACT INFORMATION IN AN EMERGENCY?

Simple ways to protect your family BEFORE a disaster strikes.

If you knew that spending 15 minutes right now could save the people you love in the event of an emergency, would you do it?

Of course you would!

During disasters like Hurricane Katrina and terrorist attacks like the London bombings, one need has come to the forefront more than any other -- the need to get a victim's identification, medical history and emergency contact information as quickly as possible. The Next of Kin Education Project, Next of Kin Registry and Shoewallet.com have joined forces to launch an international public awareness initiative, featuring ten easy ways anyone can safeguard their family in the event of a life-threatening situation.

AT HOME

You spend all your time taking care of others... But what about you? If someone had to locate your contacts in a medical emergency, could they do it? Grab your address books (we know you have more than one!), your smartphone, Outlook, Filofax and anything else you usually use and let's get organized.

First, let's create a list of emergency information for each member of the family including:

1) Their name, age, address, phone number

2) The name of their primary physician

3) Allergies and any prescription drugs the person is taking

4) Chronic medical conditions and, anything else you would want an emergency physician to know.

5) At least three emergency contacts for each person:

• For yourself, list your spouse's home, cell and work numbers, for your spouse, list your numbers. For your children, both you and your spouse's numbers.

• Next for each person, the name and contact numbers of a nearby relative or good friend;

• Then on each list, include the name and numbers of an out of state relative or friend. In case of regional emergency, you can often call long distance, even though you can't call locally. A distant friend can be a touch point for the entire family until communication is restored.

Make several copies of each list and place them:

• In an easy to find place near your main home phone

• Place each child's list in his permanent school record, in addition to his regular emergency card. Place your and your spouse's list in your personnel files at work with your other emergency information. If you don't feel comfortable having it in your file, consider placing it in a sealed envelope to be opened only in an emergency, or put the information on a password protected CD.

• With the person you chose to be your emergency contact.

• You can also put this list in your computer, or PDA so you have it with you in an emergency.

Don't forget to ask the people you want to use as contacts, for their permission to use them. Some people might not feel comfortable having to be relied upon in an emergency and it's better to know that now!

Every six months put a reminder in your calendar to review and update all of your emergency plans.

Once you get your own contacts in order, book some time with your parents, kids and the other people that you love, to make sure, in case of a medical emergency involving them, that a hospital knows how to contact you.

Home/Cell Phone

Clearly indicate your emergency contacts on your main telephone speed dial. Don't use the person's name, use their relationship to you, ie. "parents", "sister", "husband", "work". Then do the same thing on your cell phone. After the London bombings a paramedic came up with the idea of putting "ICE" (in case of emergency) on your cell phone, with the number of your emergency contact. You can do that on your cell or simply put in "husband" or "home" like you did above. Make sure you do the same thing on your Blackberry, laptop or anything else you usually carry.

Protecting Your Children

In the days after 9/11, 2,100 children were left in daycare because their parents had never indicated on their daycare emergency cards, who should be called, if the parents were unable to get to them to pick them up.

Choose someone you would want them to be with, until you can get to them and make sure that information is on the child's emergency list and on his school's emergency contact card.

Since children don't carry wallets or drivers licenses, make sure that you put Shoewallets on younger children (see information later in this article) and that older children have emergency information in their backpack, on their cell phone or anything else they carry with them.

EMERGENCY PLAN

Make sure each member of the family knows what to do in an emergency, especially if you can't get back home, or if your home is uninhabitable.

Appoint a special place for everyone to meet away from home, and make sure everyone knows who your out of state point of contact is, in case you need to relay messages to each other. Keep that plan with the emergency lists, in an easy-to-find place. Some families have even put their emergency plans on wallet sized cards, one for each member of the family.

Safeguarding Copies of Vital Information

As victims of Hurricane Katrina found, when you have to function after a major disaster, being without your driver's license, birth certificate, social security card or bank account numbers can be a huge problem.

Make a copy of all of your and your children's vital records and put them in bank safe deposit box or other secure place, preferably in two different locations. One of them should be in another city or state if possible.

If you're concerned about the security of hard copy documents, scan them onto a password protected CD, and store those instead of the hard copies.

AWAY FROM HOME

We don't have to tell you how many trauma patients end up in the ED after being hit by a car while crossing the street near their home or while jogging.

So carrying contact information with you while you're walking or jogging isn't just a good idea, it's as necessary as your running shoes!

Most accidents happen just a few blocks from home, just where people feel comfortable doing errands or going out for a run without their driver's license or other ID.

A Shoewallet/Go Wallet, is a small lightweight wallet you attach to your shoes, belt, or pocket holds an emergency contact card, and a license/credit card/key, guaranteeing your info is always right where you need it. We feel strongly about Shoewallets and their record at keeping people on the go safe! To read more about them and purchase them for your loved ones, at www.Shoewallet.com .

Another way to make sure hospitals and emergency personnel can find your next of kin in an emergency, is to register your contact information free of charge at the Next of Kin Registry www.nokr.org

Special Needs

If you or your family members have chronic medical conditions, you need to make your medical history and records easy to find in an emergency.

For the seniors in your life, make a plan for you and your relatives to take turns checking in with them every other day, to make sure everything is all right. It might also be a good idea to invest in an emergency monitoring system with a button they can press in case of a fall or other emergency.

For Alzheimer's patients, those with dementia or the mentally disabled you might have to use a combination of these tips. A Shoewallet would provide emergency ID in a place the patient won't be able to disturb. The Alzheimer's Association has a wonderful program called "Safe Return, which provides a bracelet and special tips in protecting patients who wander. And signing the person up on the Next of Kin Registry, gives an extra layer of protection in case they become lost or hurt.

Want to learn more?

To read more about our other books like the chaos clobbering "Get Your Stuff Together", go to: www.getyourstufftogether.com . §

The Benefits

WHAT ABOUT HIPAA?

How does the notification of family by emergency department personnel factor into the HIPAA environment

BY KELLEY WOODFIN, R.N., CPHRM

Implementation of the HIPAA Privacy Rule in April of 2003 has resulted in continued confusion on the part of emergency personnel regarding what information they can give out and to whom they can give it, when a patient is in the Emergency Department.

Answers to the following questions should help clarify the issues. This information is posted on the Department of Health and Human Services web site located at www.hhs.gov/faqs.

May a hospital (emergency department) notify a patient's family member or other person that the patient is at their facility?

Yes. The HIPAA Privacy Rule, at 45 CFR 164.510(b), permits covered entities to notify, or assist in the notification of, family members, personal representatives, or other persons responsible for the care of the patient, of the patient's location, general condition, or death.

Where the patient is present, or is otherwise available prior to the disclosure, and has capacity to make health care decisions, the covered entity may notify family and these other persons if the patient agrees or, when given the opportunity, doesn't object.

The covered entity may also use or disclose this information to notify the family and these other persons if it can reasonably infer from the circumstances, based on professional judgment, the patient doesn't object.

Under these circumstances, for example:

• A physician may call a patient's wife to tell her that her husband was in a car accident and is being treated in the ED for injuries.

• A nurse may contact the patient's friend to let him know that his roommate broke his leg, has had surgery, and is in recovery.

Even when the patient is not present, or it is impracticable because of emergency or incapacity to ask the patient about notifying someone, a covered entity can still notify family and these other persons.

It can do so when, in exercising professional judgment, it determines that doing so would be in the best interest of the patient.

> Even when the patient is not present, or it is impracticable because of emergency or incapacity to ask the patient about notifying someone, a covered entity can still notify family and these other persons.

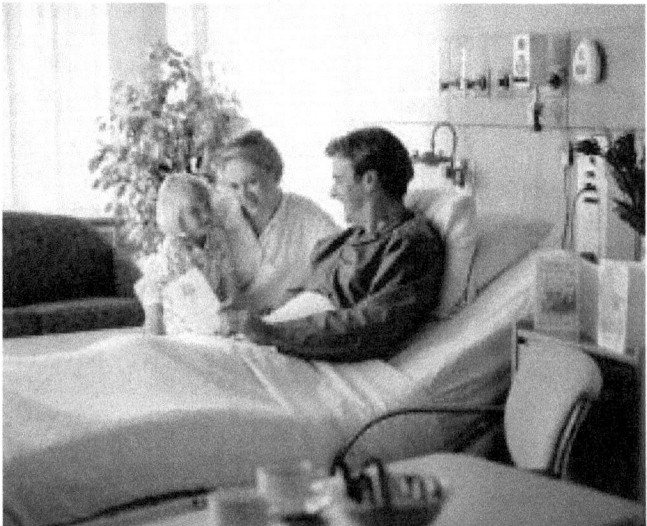

For example, a physician may, using his or her professional judgment, call the adult daughter of an incapacitated patient to inform her that her father suffered a stroke and is in the intensive care unit of the hospital.

May a hospital inform callers or visitors of a patient's location and general condition in the Emergency Department?

Yes. The Privacy Rule permits covered entities to maintain more than one type of patient directory, and to maintain multiple versions of them, provided that the other requirements at 45 CFR 164.510(a) also are followed.

For instance, Emergency Departments that maintain directory information, even though separate from or in a form different than the hospital directory of admitted patients, may still disclose the information consistent with the requirements of the Privacy Rule.

In all these cases, state law relative to patient confidentiality must also be reviewed to determine whether it is stricter that the Privacy Rule. In the event that it is stricter, state law will prevail over the Privacy Rule. For example, in the state of California, patient confidentiality statutes identify certain medical conditions and their evaluation and treatment as having greater confidentiality than all other medical conditions, such as in the case of sexual assault, substance abuse, and mental health evaluation and treatment. In these cases in California,

express written authorization from the patient must be obtained before any information can be released. Nonetheless, the provisions of 45 CFR 164.510(b) apply to the extent that the patient is not able to give consent for notification in these cases, and in the professional opinion of the medical provider, it would not be harmful to the patient to have family, personal representatives, or others notified of their whereabouts and condition.

Health professionals who have questions about this information or other provisions of the HIPAA Privacy Rule are encouraged to contact their facility's legal counsel for specific advice on compliance under the Rule in specific instances. §

At TheTone

How to leave a family & HIPAA-friendly phone message

You find your unconscious patient's emergency contact number and dial it to make the notification – only to find yourself talking to an answering machine. Now what? You have no idea who's going to pick up the message. It could be a friend, a neighbor or even a child. How do you keep from divulging private information, or worse frightening someone unnecessarily?

First of all this call is only meant to get the recipient to call you back, not to repeat information about the patient. Use a message that's simple and straightforward like this: "This is Mary Johnson at Care Central Hospital. We need to talk to Joe Smith, right away, so please have him give me a call as soon as possible at the following number." By using this simple script, your notification messages will be HIPAA and family friendly.

But what if you do reach the right person and they immediately begin to panic! Our favorite advice is from Cathleen Shanahan of Children's Memorial Hospital. "When I have to make a notification call I'll begin by telling the person on the phone who I am and ask them how they are related to the child. If it's the mom or dad, I'll tell them that their child has been brought to Children's Memorial Hospital. Of course the parent will immediately ask how the child is. This is always the hardest part of the call. If the child is clearly fine, I'll say "Don't worry, they're fine, we just need you to come down here." But if there is a more serious injury, or if the child hasn't survived, I tell them that the child has been in an accident, that they need to come down, and if necessary, that we need to get their medical history. If they refuse to get off the phone until they find out what's wrong, I'll say that we're very concerned about their child's health and that they need to come down right away. I always try to calm the person down as much as I can – tell them to go and get a pencil and paper to take down the address of the hospital, to take down my name and my number. I tell them to ask for me right away when they get here so they don't have to waste any time at the desk and then try to make sure they have someone to drive them over. I also remind them that they need to drive carefully and slowly and to make sure that they get there in one piece! " Keeping everyone in the family safe. Now _that_ is great advice!

RISK MANAGEMENT: THE IMPORTANCE OF CONTACT

Notification from a Risk Manager's perspective

BY KELLEY WOODFIN, R.N., CPHRM

From both the layperson's perspective and that of Risk Managers who have to reckon with the anger and allegations of poor service, getting a patient's family contact information must be an immediate goal of health care providers.

In emergencies, both field emergency personnel and Emergency Department staff will greatly benefit the patient if they make every effort to ensure that family is contacted as soon as practicable. When there is an emergency involving a loved one, there is nothing more critical and important to family than to be contacted and told EARLY in the situation, that their loved one is in the Emergency Department in need of care. And yet, the very nature of the E.D. conspires against staff making early contact with family or significant others who know the patient well.

Imagine, if you will, that it is your spouse, parent, or child lying in a strange environment with strangers all around, many perhaps in strange uniforms and masks, with little time to hold a hand, talk soothingly, or wipe a brow. It isn't that ED staff doesn't care; it simply is that their focus is on stabilizing the individual. Many staff members do indeed take time to speak to the patient and soothe them, but they generally can't continue to do that, for more than a few seconds at a time. Besides, there is truly nothing as comforting as having a family member at your side when you're a patient caught in the turbulence of ED evaluation and treatment.

Of course, there are many times where an individual might not have any identification on their body when they are brought into an Emergency Department. Or perhaps they may not be English-speaking, or they may be very young or very elderly, or confused by disease or injury.

In any of these circumstances, the patient may not able to give information about who to contact. Yet it is in precisely these circumstances that it is most crucial for family to be able to be with the injured or ill person, to lend comfort, and to provide emotional support. Further, the older patient may have an advance directive, or a durable power of attorney for health care wherein a designated agent is the surrogate decision-maker, and if family is not notified in a timely manner, the individual's wishes might not be carried out.

There is much greater chance of dissatisfaction and litigation in cases where family and/or significant others are not contacted and have no opportunity to participate in the person's care decisions and to comfort them. Parents are particularly susceptible to heightened anxiety and fear about their child's well-being, and become difficult to handle when they learn too late of their child's location and physical condition. In particular if the child dies before they arrive, struggles with guilt may be long-lasting and debilitating.

In other health care areas, such as long term care, most commonly family contact information is on file in the individual's record. In this area, whenever a person's condition changes, family or surrogate decision-makers need to be notified. It's the law in most states. The problem is that, not infrequently, family or surrogates are not notified in a timely manner, if at all, when a resident's condition changes. It just isn't thought about.

Yet in these cases, the resident is generally elderly and often suffers from some degree of organic brain syndrome. As a result, they might not be able to speak for themselves or make decisions about their care. Moreover, they become frightened and more confused by strange surroundings if they are sent to the hospital, and would benefit greatly from having loved ones with them.

Many of the problems associated with failure to notify or delay in notifying next-of-kin can be avoided. All nurses and physicians have to do, is direct special effort toward obtaining family contact information, or toward contacting family right away when this information is available from the patient or contained in their belongings. If no information is with the patient or they are unable for some reason to provide contact information, request assistance from the police department. In some cases, social services staff may be available to begin the search or to make the contact with family. Whatever resources are available or can be commandeered, should be tapped as soon as possible for assistance.

Remember, the person in need might be you some day, and you will want your loved ones with you as soon as possible. Teach the public to carry contact information with them at all times. Put up notices to remind them that contact information is as important as the names and doses of medications they are on. If you have an opportunity to provide a public service spot in the media, to teach the public how important it is to carry identification and family contact information on their person at all times, do it! You may be saving someone from a lot of pain and fear, and promoting quality care, all in a five minute public service spot!

Whatever you can do to ensure that family and/or significant others are contacted on behalf of a patient, make sure you make it a priority. §

reducing liability

BUT OUR HOSPITAL ALWAYS DOES THE RIGHT THING

The next time an unconscious patient comes through your ED doors, will your staff know how to keep your facility free of unnecessary liability

Recently, there was a story on the nightly news about a man who was admitted to a community hospital in critical condition after being involved in an accident on the way home from work. He died a day or two later. His family was frantic. They had no idea why he hadn't returned home. After calling everyone they could think of, friends, his co-workers and then the police, they began to call hospitals including the hospital he'd been taken to, to no avail. Five days later, they found out that he'd been in that hospital's morgue the whole time. The hospital hadn't "had a chance" to notify them that he'd been admitted or that he'd died.

In a similar case a young woman was brought into an emergency room in a compromised mental state. The hospital neglected to obtain her medical history from the hospital's own records, or phone her family for information, as she requested. Despite her objections, they refused to admit

her because they assumed she was uninsured. The woman committed suicide hours later. Her family won one of the largest jury verdicts ever given.

As much as we all hope that cases like that are unusual, they aren't. Although those are worst case scenarios, with a 16% increase in overall emergency department admissions last year, and the growing number of uninsured patients, emergency rooms are only going to get busier, stretching physicians and nurses to the breaking point. As the time trauma staffs can spend with patients decreases, so does everything that's not perceived as life saving treatment – including locating and calling the patient's next of kin. But busy as your facility is, it's still held accountable – whether by statute or by its duty to provide reasonable care, to notify your unconscious patient's next of kin or surrogate decision maker promptly. In a recent update, the Code of Federal Regulations makes an effort to deal with this problem.

42 Code of Federal Regulations 482.13(b)(4), reads as follows: "The patient has the right to have a family member or representative of his or her choice and his or her own physician notified promptly of his or her admission to the hospital."

Unfortunately the regulation doesn't contain any specific requirements about timeframes, nor does it directly address the hospital's responsibility for locating that family member or representative.

On the state level, the majority of Health Departments feel that health care providers can safely follow the practice validated by years of medical custom and social acceptance, of turning to an incapacitated patient's spouse, parents, adult children, or other close relatives as surrogate decision makers.

This practice works as long as it is followed and enforced. But that's the key. Hospitals need to follow and enforce the practice for it to work. Regulations vary considerably from hospital to hospital and even when hospitals do have well-constructed policies for notifications, they aren't always adhered to. In fact, all of the hospitals cited, had documented regulations regarding notification. As you can see from our examples of what can go wrong, a patient's family can be a vital link in his care.

Earlier we saw in Elaine Sullivan's case that one phone call to notify her daughter that she had been hospitalized, would have saved her life. Not only would her family have been able to be with her, they would have demanded that her tube feedings

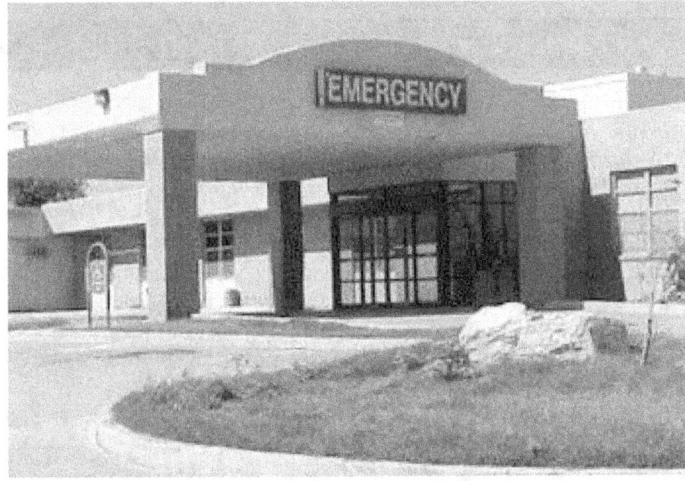

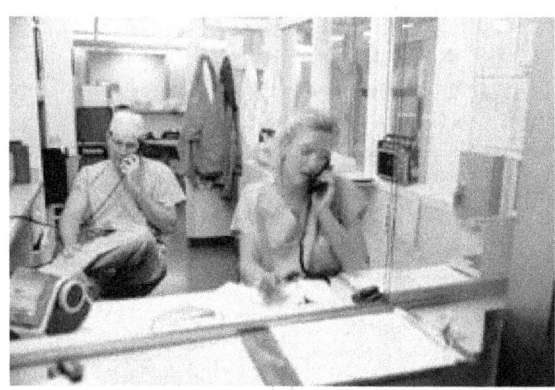

reducing liability

had taken place, that her insulin and other medications be given, and the wounds from her fall and infection treated, or they would have immediately transferred her to another hospital. Our country already believes that the families of incapacitated patients have the right to a say in their medical care. We'd like to think that we can take that one step farther – the right to be present with their loved ones during what could be the final days of their lives.

As medical professionals we have to realize that in any of those examples, that same phone call would have saved that hospital an enormous amount of liability, not to mention time, resources and potentially millions of dollars.

But how reliable are surrogate decision makers in predicting their loved one's choices for medical care versus the patient's own personal physician?

Dr. Peter Terry MD, Thoracic Surgeon and clinical professor at Johns Hopkins Medical School, asked three hundred patients to imagine three scenarios. "The best match-up between patient preferences and families' intuition of those preferences occurred with the first scenario, which shows a 70-80% accuracy of prediction. Physicians, not unexpectedly are... less accurate than family members at predicting what patients would want."

An article by Randall F. Moore, MD, JD Assistant Professor of Psychiatry, Texas A&M University, also addresses the subject. "In medical malpractice law, "informed consent" means that the physician provided sufficient information and the patient expressed a choice, either consenting to or refusing the proposed intervention.

…in some such cases, if the provider fails to adequately assess the patient's capacity and permits the patient to make an incompetent choice, the provider might be held liable, for example, for violating the patient's civil rights."

There is no way to know precisely how many people end up each year in emergency rooms, unconscious or unable to give informed consent. According to the American Hospital Association, during the last fiscal year, there were approximately 50 million "necessary" ER visits in America. Senior citizens, the group most likely to end up in the hospital in an

incapacitated state, are 39 million strong in this country. The U.S. Census Bureau officials estimate that by 2030, that number will nearly double to 76 million.

When a patient is unconscious, the practice of turning to a surrogate decision maker can seriously reduce a doctor's and hospital's risk of professional liability.

Family members can be a valuable source of information of the patient's medical history as well as his preferences for medical care. So the next time you pick up the phone to call a patient's family, don't think of it as just another duty, think of it as good medicine. §

CAN FAMILY CONTACT REDUCE PATIENT STRESS?

QUICK TIPS

To many people, the word family may not equal stress relief! But studies confirm that this is just not so. A study by Karen Grewen PhD, School of Medicine University of North Carolina, Chapel Hill, recently found that something as simple as hugs and contact with the people we love, reduces the damaging physical effects of stress. In one interesting part of the study, volunteers who were about to give speeches before large audiences, were split into two groups. One group had no contact with their spouses before the speech, while the other received hugs and well wishes from their spouses. During the speech, those that didn't receive contact's heart rates and BPs soared on average of twenty-four points more than the other group. For patient's whose stress level during trauma and illness is already high, contact with the people they love may provide the calming influence necessary to begin to reduce stress, stabilize vitals, and begin the healing process.

NOTIFY IN

7

How To Locate An ICE Contact On Your Patient's Smartphone

Written By

JANET GREENWALD

&

LAURA GREENWALD

Published by Stuf Productions/Lion And The Rock Entertainment

Table Of Contents

The Three Main Types of Smartphones

If your patient has a smartphone, changes are very good that it will be one of these three types of phone...

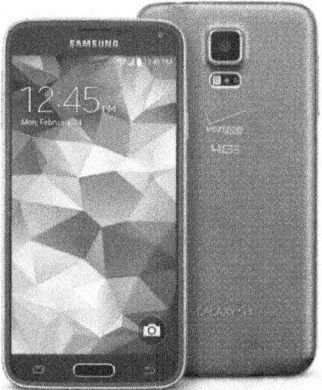

Android Phone
(Like The Samsung Galaxy)

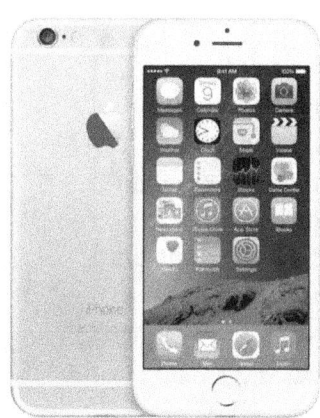

iPhone

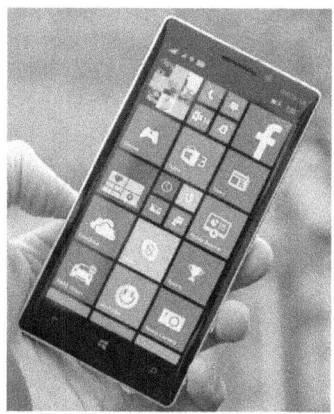

Windows Phone

But I Already Know How To Use A Smartphone... Why Are We Covering Something So Basic?

Of course you do – especially your own phone. But that doesn't mean that you're familiar enough with the other types of phones to flip them on and find your patient's ICE Contact quickly and easily.

Besides the best thing about technology is also the worst thing. How quickly it can change, morph or be completely reconfigured with the next update. Just ask the owners of the new iPhone.

You're too busy to have to figure all of that out, especially when your patient's life is hanging in the balance. So here's a little cheat sheet on the three most popular models and operating systems for the busiest people in the world – Emergency Department Personnel.

Over the next few pages you'll learn how to:
- **Turn each type of phone on**
- **Navigate the screen and open and close apps**
- **Find and use your patient's ICE Contacts or Next Of Kin**
- **And if necessary, you'll learn steps to unlock a password protected phone.**

Notify In 7

The Basics   Power On & Navigating The Screen

Power On   1

To turn on a smartphone, press and hold the power button until the screen lights up.

Power buttons can be in many different places on Android phones, but most of them are either on the upper right hand side of the phone (as it is on the Samsung Galaxy) or the top right side of the phone (as it is on the Droid Incredible).

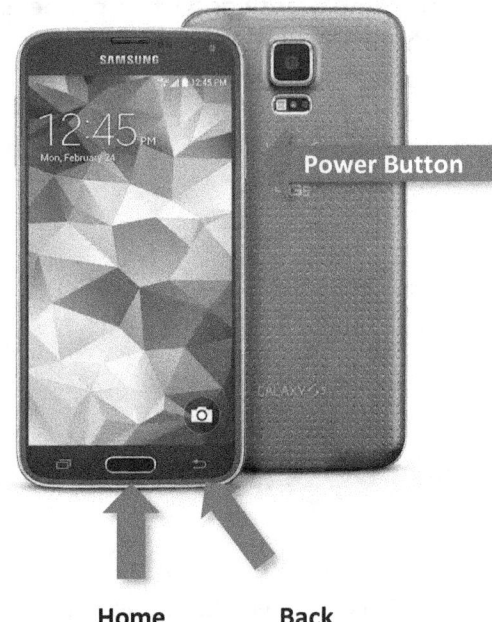

Power Button

Home   **Back**

Navigating The Screen   2

There are only three buttons you need to know to navigate around the screen of an Android phone.

The Home Button: Usually shaped like a house, this button will take you back to the home screen.

The Back Button: Usually shaped like an arrow, this button closes the app you're currently using.

The Display Apps Button: This button displays all of the Apps (applications) available on the phone. It's handy for searching for and quickly locating apps, like your patient's Contacts.

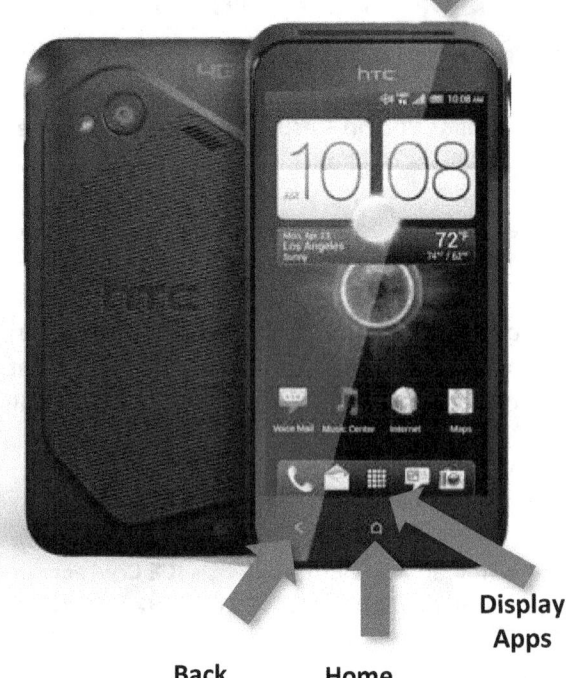

Power Button

Display Apps

Back   **Home**

4

The Basics

Navigating The Lock Screen

What Are We Looking For?   3

When you pick up a smartphone and turn it on, it will usually display the lock screen. Some users set a password to keep other people from using their phone and others do not.

So take a moment to touch the screen. If it doesn't ask you for a password, swipe the phone with your finger from left to right, to see if it will open up the home screen. If there is a little lock on the screen, place your finger in the lock and drag it to the right or left to open it.

Did the phone open? If it did, skip to Section 5. If not, continue below.

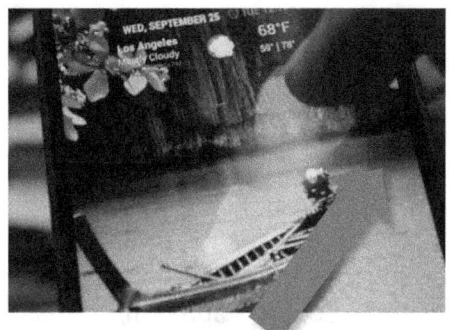

Swipe up from left to right to open

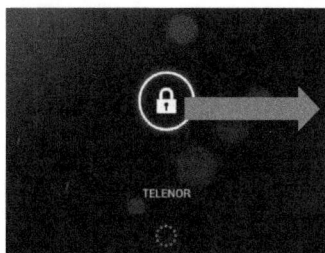

Drag the circle to the left or right to open

If The Phone Is Password Locked...   4

More and more, phone manufactures are including emergency call buttons on the lock screens of their phones. So if the phone you are holding is asking you for a password, see if you can find an Emergency Call button on the screen. If you find one, click on it to see if your patient has set up ICE Contact information or has programmed any emergency numbers into it.

No Emergency Call button? Take a look at the lock screen to see if your patient has put ICE information on their lock screen, like the example to the right. If not, you'll have to search for other ways to locate your patient's Next of Kin. You'll find tips and other strategies at the end of this guide.

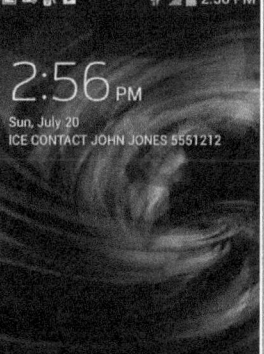

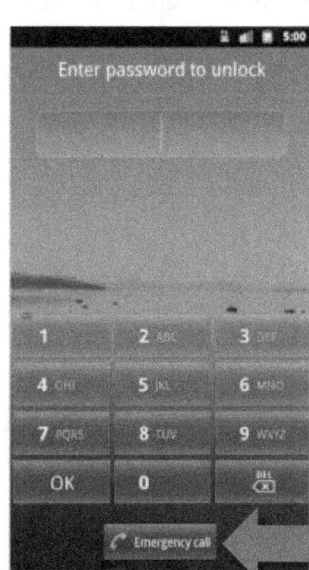

The Basics

Locating Your Patient's ICE Contacts

Finding Your Patient's Contacts

5

On the Home Screen you'll find a few ways to open up your patient's contacts. The easiest is locating the Contacts Icon and touching it to open the Contacts app. Unfortunately not everyone puts their Contacts right on their home screen.

If you can't find it, you can also touch the Phone Icon. Some phones keep the contacts list in there as well – or you can touch the Apps Icon and look for Contacts on the list of apps. They're usually listed alphabetically.

Once you find your patient's contacts, look for any designated ICE Contacts. If there aren't any, try and find his or her spouse, parents, children or any other next of kin.

If not, you'll find tips and other strategies to locate your patient's next of kin at the end of this guide.

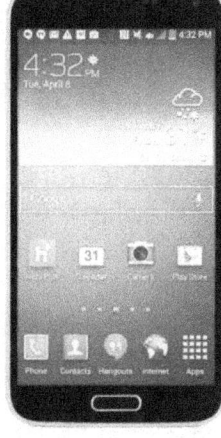

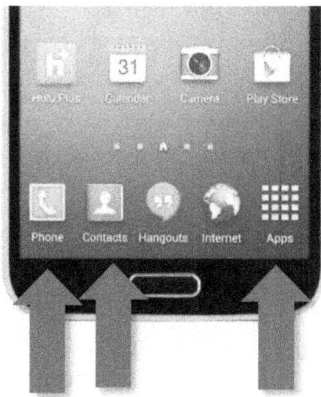

The Basics

Power On & Navigating The Screen

Power On 1

To turn on an iPhone, press and hold the power button until the screen lights up.

All iPhones (as well as iPod Touch and iPads) have the power button on the top right side – that is except for the new iPhone 6. You'll find the instructions for the iPhone 6 and 6 plus in the next section.

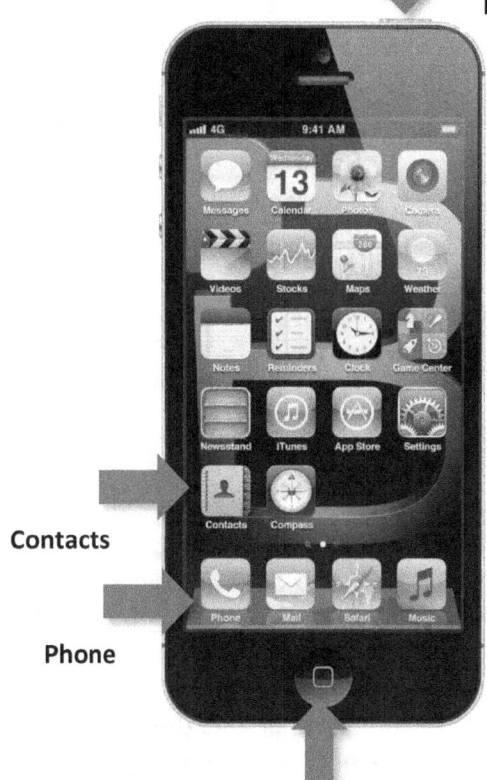

Power Button

Contacts

Phone

Home

Navigating The Screen 2

To open the phone, slide the arrow to the right to unlock.

To open an app, just touch the icon for that app, just like the Contacts app or the Phone app in the graphic above.

To close an app, double click the home key and swipe the app screen straight up until it disappears from the screen.

If the phone times out and goes back to the lock screen, just click on the home button and slide the slider bar to the right, to wake it up.

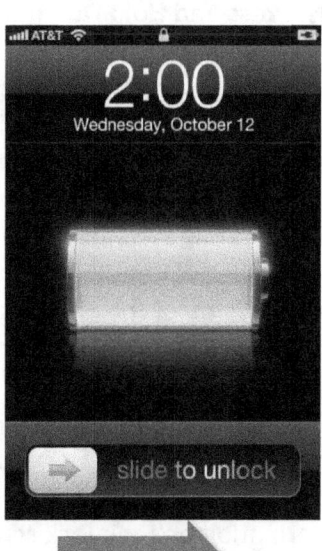

The Basics

Navigating The Lock Screen

What Are We Looking For?

3

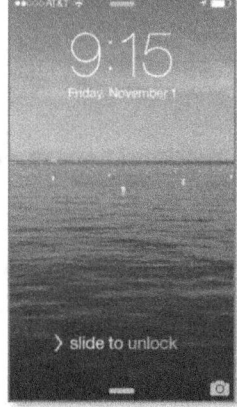
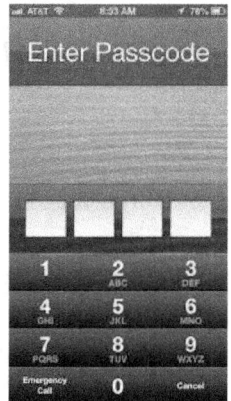

When you pick up a iPhone and turn it on, it will display the lock screen. Take a moment to touch the screen. If it doesn't ask you for a password, simply swipe the arrow with your finger from left to right, to see if it will open up the home screen. Did the phone open? If it did, skip to Section 5. If not, continue below.

If The Phone Is Password Locked...

4

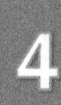

No problem. Just have a little talk with Siri! Siri is the voice activated assistant on many iPhone models, designed to help users do many tasks by voice – including looking up their contacts. The best part is, even if the iPhone is password locked, you can still get Siri's help.

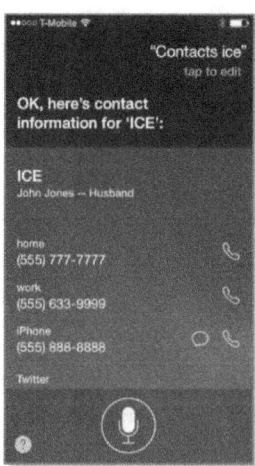
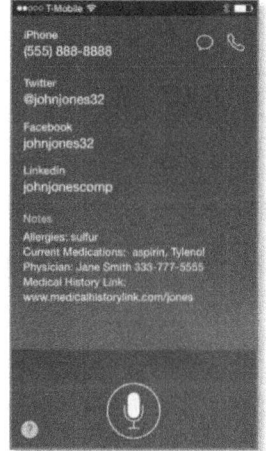

Just **Press and Hold Down** the **Main Home Key** on the phone to access Siri. Wait until Siri speaks to you and then say, "**Contacts iCE**". Siri will then display all the information the patient has saved as iCE, just like the example to the right. This won't work on some iPhones, depending on the operating system. By the way iPhone 6's work a bit differently, so if the power button is on the right side of the phone, go to the next section of this guide for instructions.

If the patient doesn't have a Siri enabled iPhone or Siri can't find an ICE Contact, look at the lock screen to see if your patient has put ICE information on their lock screen, like the example to the right.

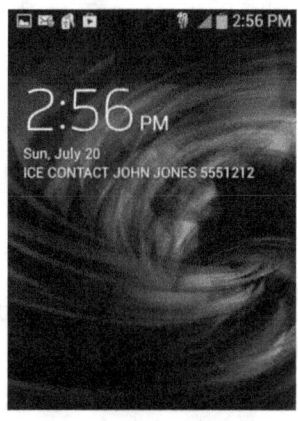

The Basics

Locating Your Patient's ICE Contacts

Finding Your Patient's Contacts

5

On the Home Screen you'll find two ways to open up your patient's contacts. The easiest is locating the Contacts Icon and touching it to open the Contacts app. Unfortunately not everyone leaves their Contacts right on their home screens.

If you can't find it, you can also touch the Phone Icon and once it opens, look at the list of contacts that are listed inside.

Once you find your patient's contacts, look for any designated ICE Contacts. If there aren't any, try and find his or her spouse, parents, children or any other next of kin.

If not, you'll find tips and other strategies to locate your patient's next of kin at the end of this guide.

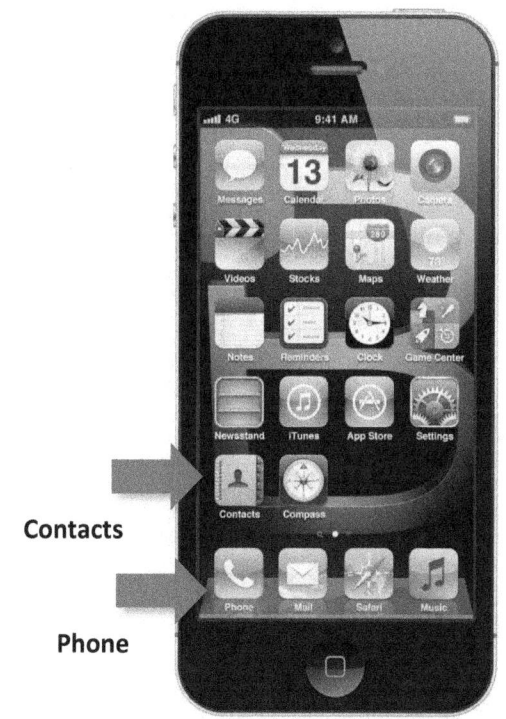

Contacts

Phone

The Basics

Power On & Navigating The Screen

Power On 1

To turn on an iPhone, press and hold the power button until the screen lights up.

On the iPhone 6 and 6 Plus you'll find the power button on the right side of the phone.

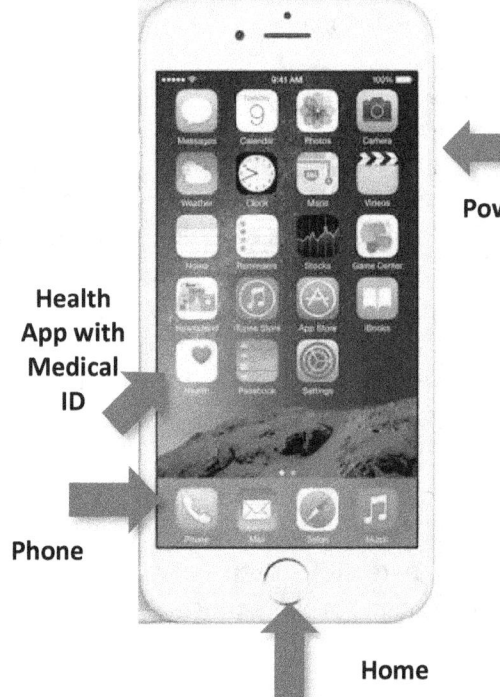

Power On

Health App with Medical ID

Phone

Home

Navigating The Screen 2

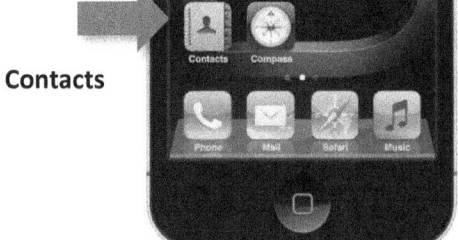

Contacts

To open the phone, slide the arrow to the right to unlock.

To open an app, just touch the icon for that app. For example, the Contacts app or the Phone app in the graphic above.

To close an app, double click the home key and swipe the app screen straight up until it disappears from the screen.

If the phone times out and goes back to the lock screen, just click on the home button and slide the slider bar to the right, to wake it up.

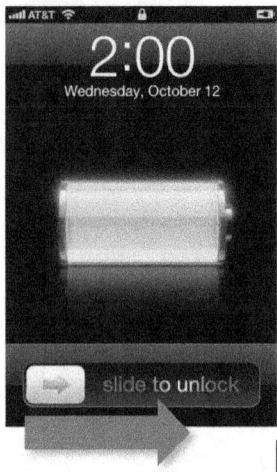

The Basics

Navigating The Lock Screen

What Are We Looking For?

3

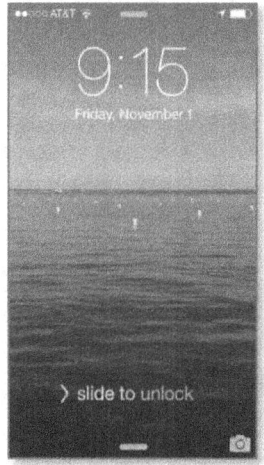

When you pick up a iPhone and turn it on, it will display the lock screen. Take a moment to touch the screen. If it doesn't ask you for a password, simply swipe the arrow with your finger from left to right, to see if it will open up the home screen.

Did the phone open? If it did, skip to Section 6. If not, continue below.

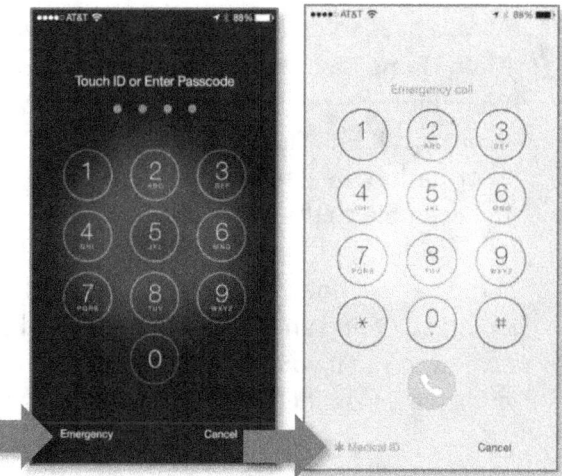

If The Phone Is Password Locked Pt. 1

4

The iPhone 6 and 6 Plus come with something no other iPhone has ever had – built in Medical ID. Even when the iPhone is password locked, if your patient has set up his Medical ID, you'll be able to retrieve it with the touch of two buttons.

On the bottom left hand side of the lock screen is the word Emergency.

Just touch it and on the screen that follows, touch the word Medical ID. This will open up the phone user's Medical ID, which should be filled with your patient's medical and vital information, or his ICE Contact information or emergency numbers. If not, there's one more thing you can try...

The Basics

Navigating The Lock Screen

If The Phone Is Password Locked Pt. 2

5

What if your patient didn't set up a Medical ID? He might still have set up an ICE Contact. And there's a way that you can find it, even with a locked phone. Just have a little talk with Siri!

Siri is the voice activated assistant on many iPhone models, designed to help users do many tasks by voice – including looking up their contacts.

All you have to do is **Press and Hold Down** the **Main Home Key** on the phone to access Siri. Wait until Siri speaks to you and then say to Siri, "**Contacts iCE**". Siri will then display all the information the patient has saved as iCE, just like the example to the right.

If the patient doesn't have a Siri enabled iPhone or Siri can't find an ICE Contact, look at the lock screen to see if your patient has placed ICE information on it like the example the right.

If not, you'll have to search for other ways to locate your patient's Next of Kin. You'll find tips and other strategies at the end of this guide.

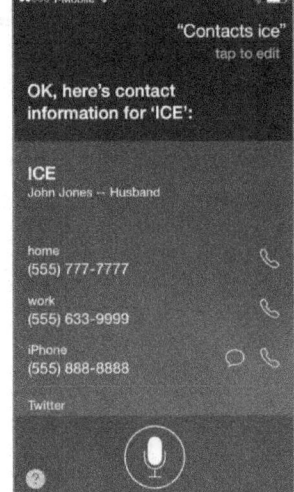

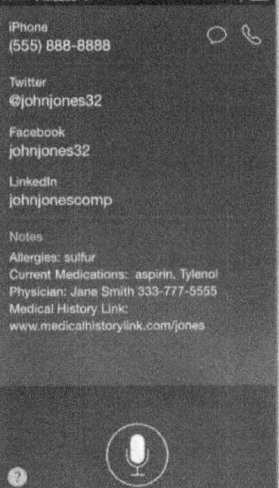

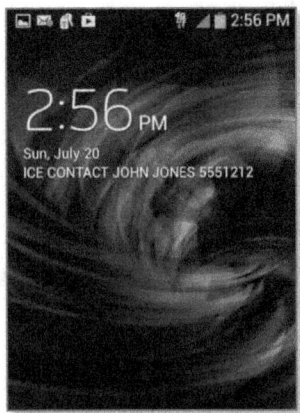

The Basics

Locating Your Patient's ICE Contacts

Finding Your Patient's Contacts

6

On the Home Screen you'll find two ways to open up your patient's contacts. The easiest is locating the Contacts Icon and touching it to open the Contacts app. Unfortunately not everyone leaves their Contacts right on their home screens.

If you can't find it, you can also touch the Phone Icon and once it opens, look at the list of contacts that are listed inside.

Once you find your patient's contacts, look for any designated ICE Contacts. If there aren't any, try and find his or her spouse, parents, children or any other next of kin.

If not, you'll find tips and other strategies to locate your patient's next of kin at the end of this guide.

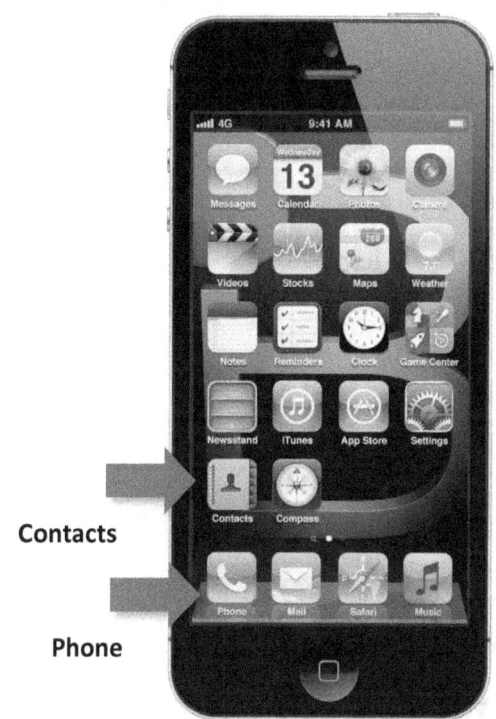

Contacts

Phone

The Basics   Power On & Navigating The Screen

Power On   1

To turn on a smartphone, press and hold the power button until the screen lights up.

The power button on the Windows phone is on the right side of the phone.

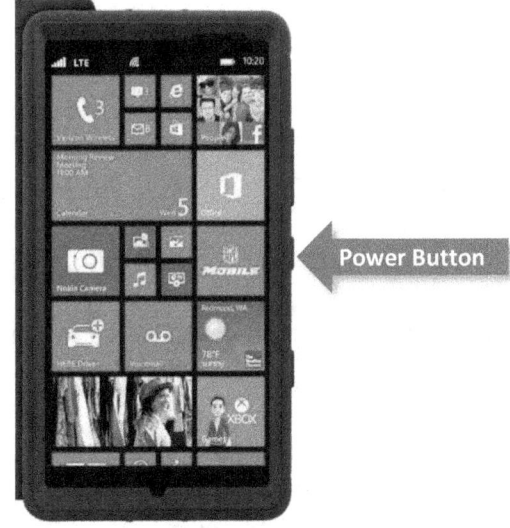

Power Button

Navigating The Screen   2

There are only two Tiles you need to know to navigate around the screen of an Windows phone.

The People/Contacts Tile: Usually is a large square with a number of pictures of different people on it, or it might also just say Contacts or People.

The Phone Tile: It has a picture of a phone handset on it.

Windows phones are highly configurable, so the app tiles you are looking for might look different depending on the phone. So we've shows a few different configurations.

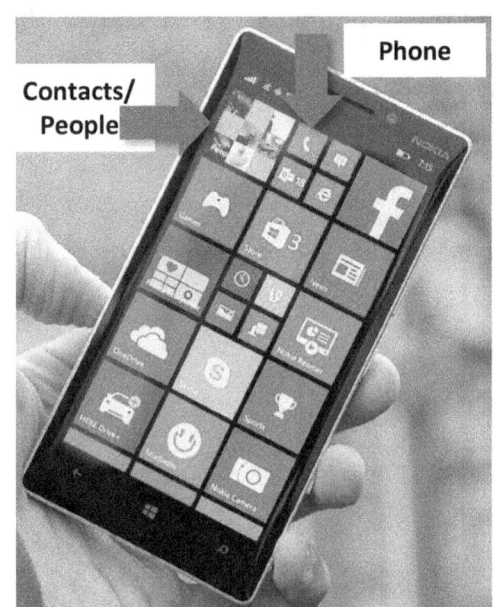

Phone

Contacts/ People

The Basics

Navigating The Lock Screen

What Are We Looking For?   3

When you pick up a smartphone and turn it on, it will usually display the lock screen. Some users set a password to keep other people from using their phone and others do not.

So take a moment to touch the screen. If it doesn't ask you for a password, simply swipe the phone with your finger from left to right, to see if it will open up the home screen. If there is a little lock on the screen, place your finger in the lock and drag it to the right or left to open it.

Did the phone open? If it did, skip to Section 5. If not, continue below.

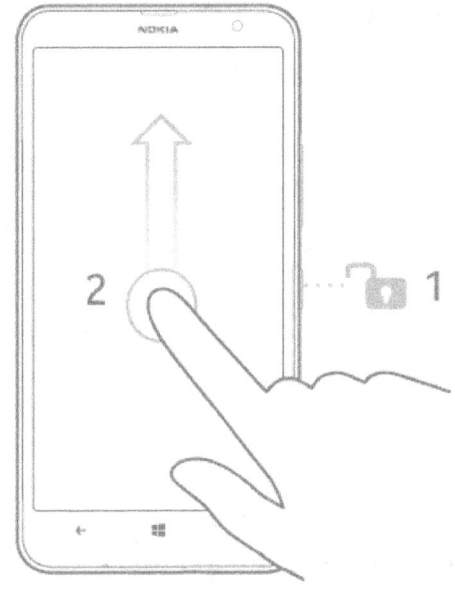

Swipe up to open

If The Phone Is Password Locked...   4

More and more, phone manufactures are including emergency call buttons on the lock screens of their phones. So if the phone you are holding is asking you for a password, see if you can find an Emergency Call button on the screen. If you find one, click on it to see if your patient has set up ICE Contact information or has programmed any emergency numbers into it.

No Emergency Call button? Take a look at the lock screen to see if your patient has put ICE information on their lock screen, like the example to the right. If not, you'll have to search for other ways to locate your patient's Next of Kin. You'll find tips and other strategies at the end of this guide.

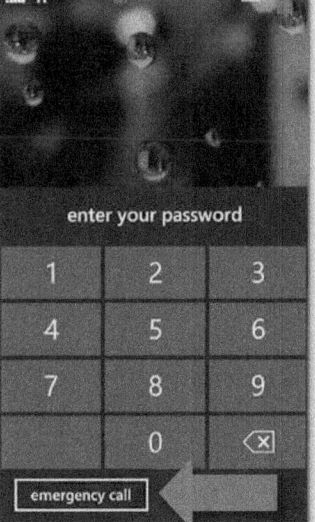

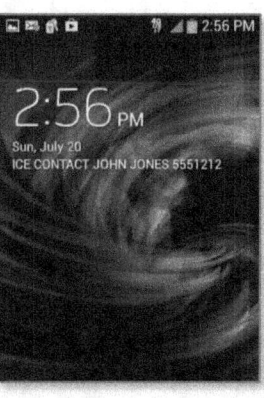

15

The Basics

Locating Your Patient's ICE Contacts

Finding Your Patient's Contacts

5

On the Home Screen you'll find a few ways to open up your patient's contacts. The easiest is locating the Contacts/People Tile and touching it to open the Contacts/People app.

If you can't find it, you can also touch the Phone Tile to locate the contacts.

Once you find your patient's contacts, look for any designated ICE Contacts. If there aren't any, try and find his or her spouse, parents, children or any other next of kin.

If not, you'll find tips and other strategies to locate your patient's next of kin at the end of this guide.

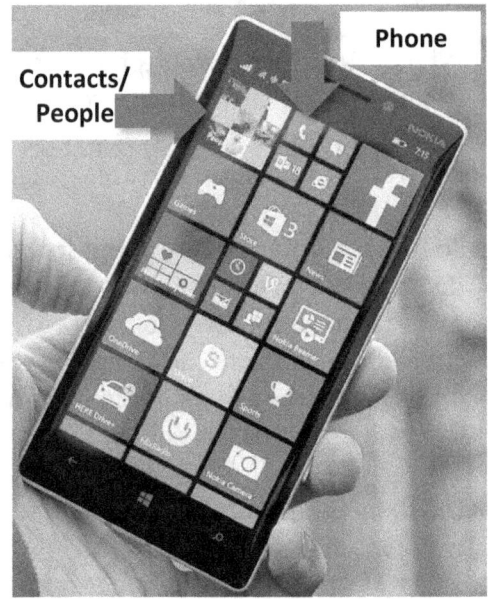

Phone

Contacts/
People

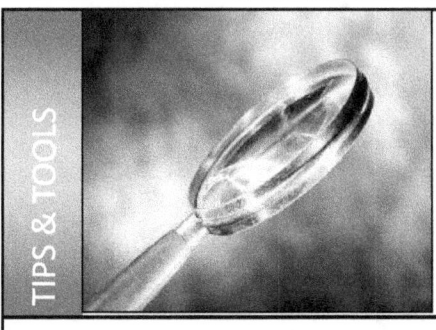

Making NOK Notifications Easier In The Emergency Department

Now that you know how to locate your patient's ICE Contacts faster and easier than ever before, here are a few other tips and tools.

- Dedicate one drawer in the ED nurse's station to all of the supplies, tracking sheets, documentation and resource material you use for Next of Kin Notification. After you put a copy of this book in the drawer, add a portable charger as well. If your patient comes in with a phone that isn't charged, or has run out of juice by the time she arrives at your door, you don't want to be wasting precious time trying to see if someone has the right charger. Portable chargers don't just charge a phone, they provide full power the instant you plug it in, so you can use it immediately. Just make sure that you choose a portable charger that comes with all the tips necessary to work with Android and Apple phones. Even better, purchase two and always keep one of them completely charged. Then the next time you encounter a dead cell phone, you can just plug it in and power it up.

- Don't forget that smartphones aren't the only electronic devices that can contain a patient's ICE Contacts. The iPod Touch, iPad, tablets and smart watches like the Samsung Galaxy and Apple Watch all have contacts, which means there might be an ICE Contact inside your patient's device. They power up and function just like their cellular counterparts, so the next time you come across a smartphone-free patient who just happens to be wearing an Android watch or sporting an MP3 player, take a look – you might just find her ICE Contact!

- Now that you know how to locate ICE Contacts, what about you and your family? Do you know how to put an ICE Contact on your phone – the right way? And yes, there is a **right** way. Don't worry though, we've got you covered. In fact, why don't you go an download a free copy of our ICE My Phone Kit at www.getyourstufftogether.com/icemyphonekit.htm while you're thinking about it. It's designed to help busy people like you put ICE Contacts on any type of phone in minutes, with all of the information necessary to communicate you and your family's specific needs in a medical emergency.

- If your facility would like a customized version of the ICE My Phone Kit to use as a value add or PR tool for your community, we'd love to create one for you. It's a great way not only to get the message out about the importance of ICE Contacts and Emergency Wallet Cards, but it's the perfect way to show your community how they can help you help them, by giving you the information you need to save their lives the next time a medical emergency strikes.

We hope you've enjoyed **How To Locate An ICE Contact On Your Patient's Smartphone** and that it makes one of the toughest jobs in the world – yours – much easier. But this guide is just a part of the **Notify In 7 System**. Notify In 7 is filled with tools that you and your staff can use to facilitate next of kin notification, patient identification and communication and everything you need to roll out the Seven Steps System facility-wide.

The book and training manual also include downloadable patient tracking workflows, tools and training materials. Notify In 7 will provide your Emergency Department staff, managers and Risk Management professionals with comprehensive training, giving you and your hospital a fully-operational Next of Kin Notification System in just 90 days.

NOTIFY IN

7

TRAINING MANUAL

Written By

JANET GREENWALD

&

LAURA GREENWALD

Published by Stuf Productions/Lion And The Rock Entertainment

Before You Begin

The Notify In 7 Training Program isn't just one book, but a collection of documents, designed to give you and your Emergency Department, ICU, CCU and Trauma staff the knowledge and tools that you need to perform notifications, identify and treat John Does, locate and use patient's medical history and enhance end of life care for patients in your facility.

Before you begin reading this book, make sure that you've downloaded all of the documents that came with it. You can download them by going to this link: www.nokep.org/notifyin7dwnld.htm and using the code NI72015 to register. Be sure to sign up right away so we can send you new resources and material updates any time they become available.

The first step in beginning your program is to familiarize yourself with Notify In 7 at the beginning of this book. Once you've read it, come back to this section book and begin the training program.

Creating Your Facility's Training Program

Now that you've read **Notify In 7**, you should:

1. Be familiar with the reasons that every hospital needs a next of kin notification program

2. Know the basics of the Seven Steps System and the way it works in a clinical setting

So how do you create, introduce and run the program in your emergency department?

Here is a breakdown of the process, designed to get you from

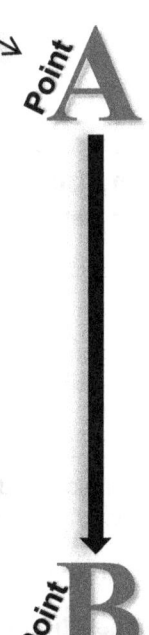

- **Assess the hospital's current NOK notification procedures, work flow and needs**

- **Analyze the current state against the ideal future (target) state. Where you are vs. where you want to be.**

- **Design a program to get from Point A to Point B**

- **Communicate the program, create tools and protocols to use while training the participants**

- **Do a pilot kick off**

- **Execute the pilot on the patient care floor**

- **Gather data on how the pilot worked**

- **Roll out the full program**

- **Create lessons learned**

- **Create a long term program plan to keep the new program working efficiently**

It's based on Six Sigma's five DMAIC phases (Define, Measure, Analyze, Improve and Control) and is a simple way to measure your progress along the way. This book is designed to be used as a workbook, so feel free to print it and write in your responses to the questions as you design your program. If you'd rather, you'll find the main questions, in the downloadable Program Workbook as well, so you can fill it in as you go, and then keep it for reference later on.

Your Current State

All hospitals have a system for notifying their patient's next of kin. The question is,

Is the system you use, right for YOUR facility?

The answer can be the difference between **life and death** for your patients and **patient satisfaction and malpractice** for you.

Maybe it's an informal system. For instance, if a patient comes into the ED unconscious, and is unaccompanied by family, the first staff member with free time, locates the patient's name and emergency numbers, calls and leaves a message with the family and if no one shows up, sends the name along to Social Service or the police. Or it could be an extremely complex system, with protocols, specified roles, responsibilities and documentation.

Your system might be ideal for a small community hospital, where everyone in town knows everyone else's family. In that case you'd probably never use John Doe procedures. But that same system would be absolutely ineffective for a major metropolitan medical center with a large homeless population.

The best part about the Seven Steps System is that it becomes the core of any hospital's notification process, no matter how simple or complex the facility's needs may be.

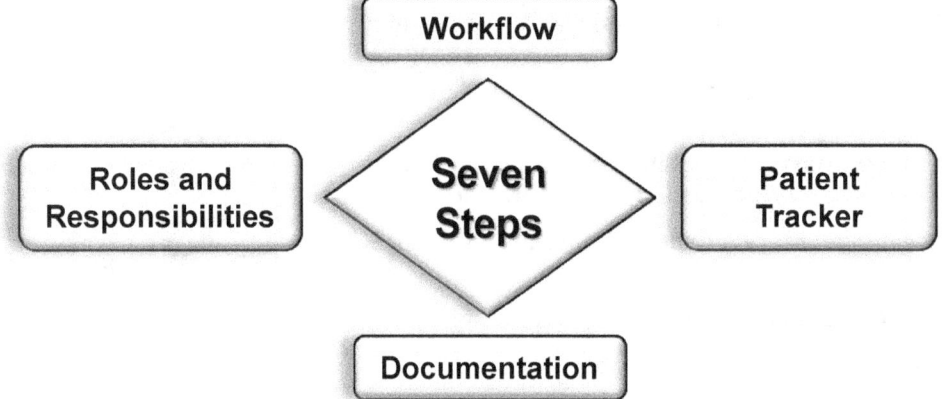

Assessment

How does your facility currently deal with patients who are in need of Next of Kin Notifications? In this section we'll help you determine what currently happens to a patient from the moment they enter your facility, until their next of kin has been notified and is on site. This way you can assess what works, what doesn't work and create the a specific program to get your staff from Point A (your current state) to Point B (the target state you desire).

What happens when an unconscious trauma patient comes rolling into your emergency department?

Seems like a simple question, doesn't it. And yet nearly every time our team poses this question to a Director of Trauma or Director of Nursing, the answer is usually embarrassed silence.

If they don't have a written work flow, (and to date only one hospital we've worked with has had one), then they begin calling their trauma team to see how the process actually works. The director of trauma or nursing talks to his or her team, and then to the triage nurses, the ED nurses, social services, pastoral care, patient advocates and sometimes even to local law authorities, just to sketch out the current work flow.

And nearly every time, that work flow is a complicated, undocumented path of procedures spanning many departments with little or no way of assessing the eventual outcome, quality of care or patient satisfaction. Worse, if the facility was ever sued and accused of failing to notify a patient's next of kin, they would have no documented way of proving that the notification actually took place.

For something this simple to track and easy to document, there is no excuse for anyone on your staff ending up in the witness box of your local courtroom!

So let's see how your facility currently performs the notification process.

If you are the head of trauma services or have an in-depth knowledge of the current process, you can begin to answer the questions below yourself, and ask staff members for their input on areas you are not familiar with. If you don't have in-depth knowledge, you'll need to find everyone who is involved in the next of kin notification workflow for your hospital, and interview them to discover who does what, when. You can either print this book out and fill in the answers by hand, or fill them in, in the Program Workbook (the .xls file in the files you downloaded).

Does your facility have a written protocol for notifying a trauma patient's next of kin?

If so, how old is it? Is this protocol followed? (You may not be able to answer this question completely until you speak to all of the staff members involved. The written protocol may be quite different from actual practice.)

How To Uncover Your Current Notification Work Flow

Let's pretend for a moment that you've just been called to the ED on a very busy afternoon, to sign off on some paperwork.

The trauma bay doors open and paramedics roll a man named Jack Johnson into the department on a gurney. He has been in an MVA, is unconscious and is unaccompanied by family. According to paramedics he is in serious to critical condition. All they found at the scene was his wallet.

Your assignment is to document everything that normally happens in your trauma department, from the moment he is rolled into the ED, until his wife arrives on scene.

Jack is transported into your ED. Who is the first person to interact with Jack and what is their title? Is this the person that makes the determination whether the hospital will need to call his next of kin or surrogate decisionmaker? If not, who does? Do they always perform that role, or do others perform it as well? If so, what are their titles?

Is there a place on your chart or any separate paperwork that your staff uses to track the progress as they locate and notify a patient's next of kin? If not, how do you document that a notification has taken place or what the status is of a notification in progress?

The staff member that is tasked with assessing your patient's status, has determined that Jack's next of kin needs to be notified. What happens next?

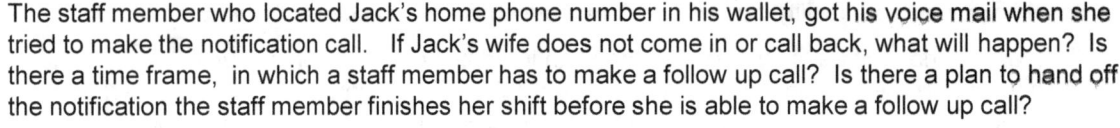
The staff member who located Jack's home phone number in his wallet, got his voice mail when she tried to make the notification call.   If Jack's wife does not come in or call back, what will happen? Is there a time frame, in which a staff member has to make a follow up call? Is there a plan to hand off the notification the staff member finishes her shift before she is able to make a follow up call?

And then what happens?

And then what happens?

And then what happens? (follow the process step by step, all the way through to completion)

What happens if the person who the staff notified, never comes in? Who does the staff hand the notification process over to? When does the handover take place? (follow the process all the way through to completion)

What if Jack doesn't have anyone at home and your trauma staff can't find any relatives? What happens? (follow the process all the way through to completion)

Now let's assume that Jack was a jogger without any identification on his body. He's now a John Doe? What procedure do you follow?

What does the trauma staff do to located his identification? Do they hand it over to a different department? Is there a process for this? Does the department that takes over have a process for identifying John Does?

Are there any times during the day or on the weekends when there is no one available to complete parts of the notification process? For example, if a John Doe is referred to social work, and no one is in the office over the weekend, a John Doe could go unidentified for 48 hours. When you create your new program, you would be able to task a different staff member take this responsibility on weekends.

Go back over the processes that you have detailed. Is there anything missing? Are there any other kinds of notifications or circumstances that your staff frequently deals with? If so, note those as well along with the current procedures and work flows. Once you're certain you have a complete picture, go on to the next section.

> ### During Define You Will:
>
> ● Use the review you completed to assess your current processes
>
> ● Define the changes you wish to make
>
> ● Form an idea of what you want your Target State to look like
>
> ● Fill the key roles on your Program Team
>
> ● Begin filling in the program worksheet

Evaluating the Current Process

Were you surprised at the answers to the questions in the last section? Were your facility's processes more detailed than you thought, or less detailed? Did you see anything that you want to change, or clarify? Are too many people involved in the process, or not enough?

Do you have criteria that determines which patients need to have their NOK notified? For example, do you call the NOK of patients who are completely unconscious and are unaccompanied by next of kin, or do you also include patients who are awake, but not oriented and cannot give informed consent?

How long does your staff currently take to perform a next of kin notification? Let's say that a patient comes in unconscious, but her next of kin is clearly noted in her cell phone. Is there a time frame, by which the first call needs to be made?

If a family member doesn't respond to the first call, do you have a time frame in when the follow up call needs to be made?

If you have a written set of protocols or processes, do your staff members follow them? Do they work? Who is in charge of updating them and how often are they updated?

In short, from your review of the entire notification process beginning to end, does your facility's process work? If not, jot down some specific notes on what doesn't work, what needs to be improved and how you would like those improvements to work.

Dealing with Special Populations

Are there specific problems that need to be addressed based on your hospital's population?

Y   N   Are you in a large metropolitan area?

Y   N   Do you have a large amount of trauma patients versus other facilities?

Y   N   Do you have a large senior citizen population?

Y   N   Do you have a large amount of patients coming in who require next of kin notifications?

Y   N   Do you have a large amount of John Does?

Y   N   Do you have a large non-English speaking population?

Are there any other needs or problems based on the needs of your patients, that you have uncovered during the review? How do you feel they need to be dealt with?

Now that you have determined how you currently perform next of kin notifications, we can move on to the next step, assigning roles for the Notify In 7 Program.

No matter how large your facility is, you really only need three or four people to create, design and execute your facility's new Next of Kin Notification Program.

Here are the roles:

Notification Program Manager (NPM)

This is the person who oversees and is ultimately in charge of the Notification Program – probably you! If not, the ideal person for this role would be the head of trauma services, emergency services or the director of nursing. The NPM works with the Trauma Notification Manager and Program Coordinator to:

> •**Review current notification practices**
>
> • **Create and Develop a customized notification program for your facility**
>
> • **Obtains management approval for and signs off on the details of the hospital's notification program**
>
> • **Assigns team members to the roles they will play during notifications**
>
> • **Oversees the TNM and Program Coordinator as they develop communications to staff members about the program's rollout, perform the program kickoff and the actual execution of the pilot and program in the emergency department.**

The role of Notification Program Manager (NPM) will be performed by:

Trauma Notification Manager (TNM)

This is the person who holds a management position within the emergency department and will be responsible for the rollout and execution of the Notification Program. The TNM works with the NPM to:

> • **Consult on the creation and development of the customized notification program for the facility.**
>
> • **Supervise team members who perform notifications, answer questions and address problems.**
>
> • **In a smaller facility, this TNM might actually perform the notification process her/himself.**
>
> • **As the pilot progresses, reports back to the NPM to discuss any changes that need to be made or report on successes.**

The role of Trauma Notification Manager (TNM) will be performed by:

Notification Program Coordinator (PC)

This is the person who is responsible for scheduling the overall timetable of the program. The PC will: set start and end dates for each of the five phases, keeping the team on task and on time, and keep track of issues and report on the final results. The PC will also gather current ED statistics from the previous year or six months (if possible) to determine the current effectiveness of procedures and set measurable goals for improvement.

> **• Set start and end dates for each of the five phases during the creation of the notification program, keeping the team on task and on time**
>
> **• Make sure that the notification team has everything that they need on the patient care floor, like the tracking notebook and worksheets and that everything is kept in order during the pilot.**
>
> **• Keep track of any issues that arise and report on the final results**
>
> **• In a large facility, the PC can gather current ED statistics from the previous year or six months (if possible) to determine the current effectiveness of procedures and set measurable goals for improvement.**

The role of Notification Program Coordinator (PC) will be performed by:

Training & Communications Coordinator

In a smaller facility this role can easily be assumed by the Trauma Notification Manager.

> **• Communicate the new processes and roles to staff members and create the documents used to train the team members who will be performing notifications.**
>
> **• Make sure that all departments are kept abreast of the changes including the ED staff, social work, risk management, pastoral care, patient advocates and anyone else who will be a part of the notification process**

The communication and kick off could take place in a half day seminar, or for a smaller facility could simply consist of a memo with a guide covering the new program and work flow, the role each person will be playing and the results that the hospital is expecting.

The role of Training & Communications Coordinator (TC) will be performed by:

You now know how your facility currently handles notifications, what works and what doesn't. But before we go on to the next phase, you'll need to know the answer to the following question.

What does your ideal notification Work Flow look like?

Just as it's impossible to drive a car blindfolded (at least if you have any hope of getting where you're going), it's also impossible to drive change, if you don't know where your destination looks like.

Here is your next exercise. Use the Target State Tab in your Program Workbook to capture the results.

Sit down for about fifteen minutes in a quiet room where you won't be disturbed. With everything that you've discovered in your own facility, close your eyes and picture Jack Johnson, the patient from the last section, coming into your ED six months from now. Visualize your ideal work flow, where everything works exactly like you want it to.

Who greets Jack? Assesses him? How is that assessment performed.

In what time frame should the notification be performed? How does your staff go about locating his personal information, or identifying him if necessary?

How do they perform the notification? Who follows up on the notification and how?

Then meet with your TPM and Program Coordinator to discuss your thoughts, get their input and define the differences between the current work flow the hospital currently uses and the target work flow you want to see instituted.

What are your expectations? What do you hope to gain from this program?

• A statistical rise in patient care satisfaction?

• Quicker response time in locating and notifying patient's next of kin?

• Better documentation every time a patient notification is made?

• Problems that need to be solved based on the hospital's patient population (John Does, Seniors, non English speaking)?

Your final assignment for Define is to work with your Program Coordinator to sketch out a time table for the program. By using the phase time table below, you can easily implement this program in 90 days. You will do the actual Pilot of the program during the Improve phase and then work out any kinks during the Control phase.

What date will you hand the new notification process over to the trauma manager to manage as part of the daily ED routines?

Record the time you are estimating for each phase and deliverable below or in the Time Table tab on the Program Workbook. Keep in mind that the time table is fluid (at least for now) and is able to be changed depending on how your pilot and program plans progress. It can always be shortened or lengthened if need be. Set regular weekly or biweekly meetings with your team as you work through each phase.

Phase	90 Day Timeframe	Your Timeframe/Dates
Define	14 Days	
Measure	14 Days	
Analyze	7 Days	
Improve/Pilot	40 Days	
Control/Assessment	15 Days	

> **During Measure You Will:**
>
> ● **Decide how the Chart Worksheet will be used and how notifications will be documented.**
>
> ● **Fill the three critical roles necessary for performing notifications on the patient care floor.**
>
> ● **Design and set up your Notification Tracking Notebook.**

Notification Team Roles and Responsibilities

No matter how large your facility is, there are only three roles that need to be performed, to provide successful next of kin notifications. Each role needs to be covered for every shift and together form the backbone of the notification process. They are:

The Assessor

The Notifier

The Follow Up

Basically, the Assessor, evaluates the patient to see if they meet the three U's. Is the patient...

Unconscious?

Unaccompanied by next of kin?

Unable to give informed consent?

If the answer is yes, then the **Assessor** starts a Patient Tracking Worksheet and pages the Notifier.

The **Notifier** searches for the patient's emergency contact info, home number, if necessary identity, makes the notification calls and follows the patient until the NOK arrives onsite or until it's established that the notification can't be made. Once the Notifier is finished he or she pages the Follow Up.

The **Follow Up** takes it from there, to use advanced means to identify the patient or find the next of kin, or to follow up after a successful notification, to ensure patient satisfaction.

On the next page you'll find an in-depth look at each position.

1. The Assessor

Ideally this role will be performed by the Triage Nurse, Nurse Manager, or a Resident – whoever normally assesses patients on arrival. Along with their normal assessment procedure, they will determine if the patient is unconscious or altered and if they are unable to give informed consent. They will then determine if the patient is alone, or is unaccompanied by next of kin or a surrogate decisionmaker. If they are unconscious, unable to give informed consent and unaccompanied by next of kin, the Assessor will begin a Seven Steps Chart Worksheet and hand the notification over to the person in the Notifier role.

2. The Notifier

The Notifier is an Emergency Department nurse or unit coordinator who gathers any information that is physically on the patient and performs the steps necessary to locate a next of kin contact or identify the patient if he/she is a John/Jane Doe. Once the contact name/number is found, the Notifier makes the notification calls and follows the case until the next of kin arrives on scene.

Once they have arrived the Notifier will greet the family and make sure that they are seen by the patient's nurse or physician. If information is not found on the patient, or if the NOK doesn't call back within the time limit on the Chart Worksheet, the patient's Chart Worksheet and information will be handed off to the Follow Up.

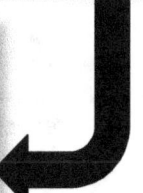

3. The Follow Up

The Follow Up person is a staff member in social services, patient advocacy or pastoral care, who has two specific duties. First, this is the person who comes on the scene if all of the Notifier's efforts to identify a patient or find a next of kin contact within the given amount of time, have been unsuccessful. The follow up person takes ownership of the patient's Chart Worksheet and other information and continues to try and locate his identity or if identified, his NOK contact for a specified period of time. If this is not successful, the patient's case is handed over to its final destination according to facility policy, depending on the patient's diagnosis and outcome.

Follow Up also receives the complete worksheets each time a notification is made to: perform quality assurance, call the family or visit the patient to ensure that everything is fine, keep the worksheets in a file to be used for reference, patient statistics, metrics or in service training.

Every facility has its own culture and its own way of splitting up the work on the patient care floor. Now that you have an idea of the roles and responsibilities of the Notification Team, how do you see each role playing out in your Emergency Department?

Do you have an idea of which job title should perform which task?

The role of Assessor will be performed by: Ex. *Triage Nurse*

The role of Notifier will be performed by: Ex. *Nurse Manager*

The role of Follow Up will be performed by: Ex. *Patient Advocate*

Patient Tracking 101

If you've been in medicine any length of time, you've already discovered making a notification is not a task, it's a PROCESS. There are just too many variables. A patient with ID, might not have any emergency contacts. A patient with contacts, might not have anyone available by phone before 6 pm. And a Jane Doe or a homeless person, might have her ID hidden or the contacts could be twenty years old.

To deal with the variables, you need a system that

A.   Follows the patient wherever he goes in your facility

B.   Will keep notification team members up to date, even if they've just come on shift and don't yet know the patient

C.   Will provide solid documentation of every step that was made to locate and notify the patient's next of kin, when it was taken and by whom, satisfying local and state requirements and reducing legal liability.

Welcome to the Notification Tracking System!

By using our simple Seven Steps Patient Tracking Worksheet, your facility can track patients from the beginning to the end of the notification process, right in the patient's chart or in a separate tracking notebook.

First you need to decide which approach will work best for your facility.

Do you have an electronic charting system, or paper based charts for your patients?

If you have paper based charts, the worksheet can be placed and used directly in the patient's chart. If you use an electronic charting system you will have to keep the worksheets in the Notification Tracking Notebook, or ask your IT department if they can create a version of the worksheet that they can integrate with your electronic charting system.

When will the worksheet be used?

Will the worksheet be included in all of your patient's charts, whether they do or don't need an NOK notification performed? Or will this only be placed into the charts of patients who need a notification.

Which version of the worksheet will work best for your facility?

Take a look at the two versions of the worksheet that were included with your program. Both have the same information, but one is in worksheet format and the other is in chart page format. Either can be filled in right on the computer screen using Microsoft Word, or by hand, on the fly, right at the patient's bedside. Decide which version will work best for your facility.

Creating the Notification Tracking System Notebook

Since most of the Notifications will take place in the Emergency Department, that's where the Tracking Notebook should reside. We'll get into the details later, but depending on your program, it will include:

- **Patient Tracking Worksheet Pages**
- **Definitions of Roles and Responsibilities**
- **The Seven Steps**
- **Your Facility's Notification Work Flow**
- **Your Notification Policies**
- **Tips on Locating Emergency Contact Information**
- **Tips on Identifying John Does**
- **Any information you wish to include on specialty notifications, like pediatric, or Alzheimer's patients.**

The Notebook should be in a place that is safe, easy for your staff to locate, yet in a place where patients, visitors or non-staff members will not be able to view it.

SEVEN STEPS TO SUCCESSFUL NOTIFICATION			PATIENT TRACKING WORKSHEET	
Patient Name:	Date:	Time Admitted to ED:		
Name of **Assessor**:	Title:	Name of **Notifier**:	Title:	

Step 1 Patient Status Confirmed

Is patient unconscious? ___Yes ___No

If the patient is conscious, is he/she physically or mentally unable to give informed consent. ___Yes ___No
Does the patient have a family member or surrogate decision maker in attendance? ___Yes ___No
If the answers to all three of these questions are yes, page **The Notifier** on duty and have them continue with **Step 2**.

Step 2 Examine Personal Effects

Examine patient's personal effects for an emergency contact number. If patient doesn't have an emergency card in his/her wallet, check the patient's purse, brief case or day planner, clothing, or cell phone for home or emergency numbers.

Was an emergency contact name found? ___Yes ___No ____Time   If yes, go to step 5. If no, go to **step 3**.

Step 3 Retrieve Patient's Home Number

If you can't find a specific person/number named as an emergency contact, try to locate the patient's home telephone number.

Home number found? ___Yes ___No ____Time   If yes, go to step 5. If no, go to **step 4**.

Step 4 Seek Other Sources For Information

Look for the patient's emergency contact information on records from his/her previous hospital admissions, or by calling his doctor's office or his insurance company.

During Define we asked you if your facility serves any other populations that need special attention in the notification process. If you identified any special populations, now is the time to decide how you want to handle them.

Do you want to design or use a special worksheet for John Does?

Do you serve a large population of Alzheimer's patients or patients who are physically or mentally challenged?

If so you might want to have Subject Matter Experts -- staff members who have special training in working with those types of patients – help design specialized workflows and oversee the notification process in those cases.

During your next meeting with your TPM and PC, and elicit their feedback as well as the feedback of anyone that you feel should have a voice in the way the Tracking System will work in your facility.

Now is a great time to begin documenting lessons learned during this process, so details won't be lost later on, as you become involved in setting up your pilot. You can track Lessons Learned in your Program Workbook.

It's also time to set up management routines to ensure that everything moves forward once the Notification Team comes on board.

For example, once the Pilot gets going, if one of the Notification Team Members has a problem with the process or comes up with a great idea, who should she go to? Will the TPM handle those things on a daily basis, or do you want team members to come directly to you with problems and feedback.

What if a team member isn't performing the function – who will step in and take care of the problem? If there are problems identified during the Pilot, how do you want them to be dealt with?

Identifying potential problems now, will help keep the Pilot rolling smoothly later!

During Analyze You Will:

○ **Create a new workflow to help you achieve your Target State**

○ **Design and set up your Notification Tracking System**

○ **Create your Pilot Plan**

Creating a Notification Workflow

The Notification Workflow is simply a chart that shows from beginning to end, the steps to:

○ Assess whether or not a patient needs to have their next of kin notified

○ Locate that emergency contact information

○ If the patient is a John Doe, obtain the patient's identity

○ Make the notification

○ Follow up to make sure the family is on site

○ If the information or identity is not located, hand the worksheet off to the department that will continue the intervention.

On the next page is the basic Notification Workflow, used by the hospitals for which we've consulted over the last few years.

As you can see, even thought it follows the same flow as the chart worksheet, it provides a detailed look at the notification process, to cover all eventualities your team will face as they perform NOK notifications.

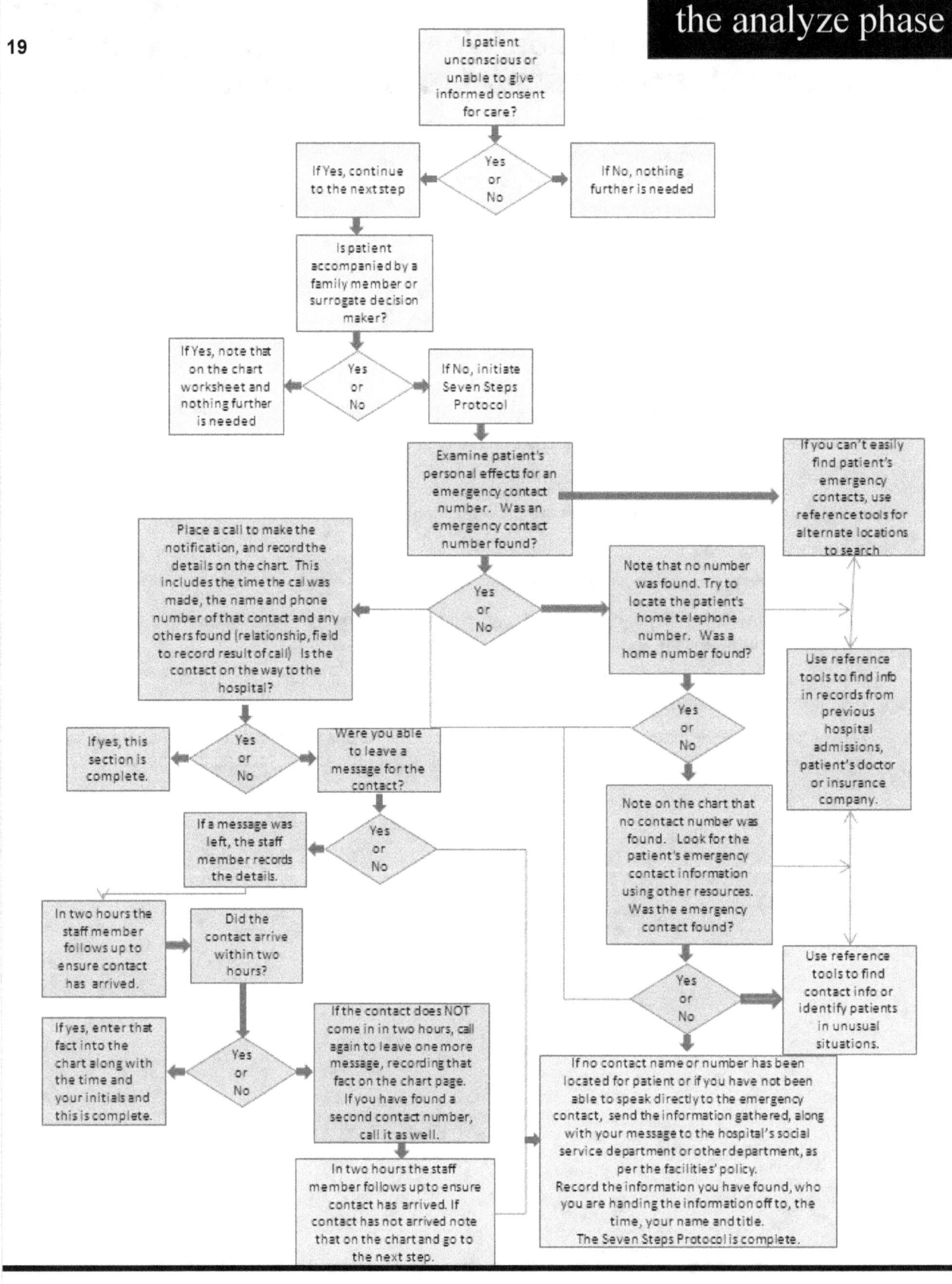

You'll notice that the squares change colors as the process progresses. That's because each square is color coded depending on which of the three team members are responsible for that task.

> **Assessor is PEACH**
>
> **Notifier is LIGHT BLUE**
>
> **Follow Up is LIGHT GREEN**

Although this process is proven to work exceptionally well for everyday notifications, your facility might have additional needs. For example you might have a large homeless or John Doe population to deal with. So you may want to design a second work flow and Chart Worksheet for unidentified patients.

In the downloads you'll find a PowerPoint document called Workflow.ppt. Here you'll find a copy of the workflow that we just showed you, but it's in PowerPoint, so you can move the pieces around any way you want, to create your own specialized workflows. Or you can keep the workflow as it is, but add in the names or titles of the team members who will be responsible for each area.

Two caveats.

1. Before you begin playing with the Workflow file, save it, with a different name to your desktop or two a flash drive, so you don't overwrite the original file.

2. If you drastically change your overall Notification Workflow to the point that tasks will be in a different order than they are on the current workflow, remember to make those same changes on the Patient Tracking Worksheet. Otherwise your team will have no idea what they're doing!

The Pilot Rollout Plan

You have your long term vision for the way you want Notifications to be performed in your facility. You know how the Seven Steps System works, you have your Workflow(s), your Patient Chart Worksheets and your Notification Tracking System Notebook.

Now it's time to get the team assembled and create your Pilot Plan.

Our first piece of advice is to keep it simple. As we said before, notification is a PROCESS. Every patient and every notification is different and I'm sure there isn't one ED professional who hasn't been surprised, upset, pleased or challenged more often than they ever expected.

For your Pilot Plan you will need:

• Your list of roles, responsibilities and the titles of the people you wish to place in those roles

• Sign off from any managers necessary

• To place your final workflow(s) and Chart Worksheet(s) in the Notification Tracking System Notebook

• Specific dates the Pilot will begin and end

• Management Routines during the Pilot (who reports to whom, how do you deal with problems, concerns, personnel problems and suggestions/procedure changes)

• Communication Plan

• Training Plan

Once you receive sign off on your Pilot plan, you can begin to put the Pilot together.

Communication Plan

Approximately one month before the Pilot, you should begin to communicate with the people that you identified to be a part of the Notification Team, as well as any other people or departments who will be affected by the change in the way patient notifications will be handled. For example, if patient advocates used to be involved with the process, but will no longer be involved, you might want to talk with the department manager to tell her about the new workflow you are using to streamline the process and the workload this will take off of her team. A little spin never hurts!

If you decided to use a Training and Communications Coordinator, now is the time to engage her/him. Invite the Coordinator to the next meeting that you hold with your TPM and PC, review the Pilot timeline and discuss the needs you are going to face as you design the communications and training plan. Here are a few questions to guide you through the process. Your TPM, will probably be the best resource for these answers since she or he already works with trauma/the ED.

Is the new notification procedure a great deal different from what your ED staff is now using?

Are the members of the new notification team familiar with performing notifications?

Do you think that they will have a hard time learning the new workflow and Chart Worksheet?

Are there people now involved with the process, who have never done notifications?

If you were to give all the new Notification Team members a copy of Notify In 7 along with handouts specifying their role and how to perform it, do you think this would suffice, or will they require more training?

Are there any problem areas the TPM or Training and Communications Coordinator can foresee in preparing the team for the Pilot?

In our experience, a series of fun, very brief communications along with a two hour training course and kickoff celebration to begin the pilot, usually work best.

With the brief communications, you're letting the team know what will soon be coming and how it will impact them. Now that you're implementing the notification system, you're actually giving them the tools they need to make a difficult part of their jobs, quicker and easier. Make sure that you communicate that. If you do the communications in such a way that you're doing a countdown to the Pilot, you're giving them something to look forward to, while preparing them, so that they'll be ready to go and know what to do, the moment the Pilot begins.

Another great thing to communicate is what everyone is going to get out of it. Here are some positives to highlight:

● Using the Seven Steps will actually be less work in the long run, because it gives your team a step by step guide in what to do, how to chart and even how to identify patients, which is usually a difficult, time consuming, emotional process.

● Training will be minimal, you're simply reinforcing what the hospital already does in NOK situations and providing a framework to fill the gaps that need to be put into practice.

● The hospital will be able to document NOK occurrences and the steps taken, to help prevent litigation. For the six NOK states, it will protect the hospital in light of the NOK law.

● It will help the hospital gather unconscious patient's medical history, drug history and get informed consent signed more quickly, giving patients better care, helping the trauma team save more lives in less time and decreasing liability in case of negative outcomes.

Along with the positives are the negatives. Just a couple that you might want to be ready to address:

● The idea that this will create more work for the team

● The learning curve

● Extra time spent reporting and training

● We already have processes in place, why change? Notifications aren't my job, that's for the police or fire department.

Your final step is to hand over the plans to the Training and Communications Coordinator so that she/he can begin designing the communications, begin sending out some Save the Date emails to the affected staff members and to set up any training sessions and Kick Off Celebrations you have decided upon.

Management Routines

Just a quick word about Management Routines.

While no hospital staff has the time or energy to attend an endless schedule of meetings, getting together on a regular basis, especially when the staff is doing something new, is vital.

We propose that the Program Manager, TPM, PC and Communications Coordinator hold bi-weekly meetings with the Notification Team during the pilot, either by holding one meeting per shift or having everyone meet at once via conference call. Don't make it more than an hour, but it's a great opportunity to touch base to see how the pilot is progressing. You can even discuss the Tracking System Notebook to see how things went with specific patients and how things are going overall. If there are problems or questions address them as a team. If there are suggestions or if there are frustrations listen carefully. And if anything is brought up that needs to be addressed by upper management or a department not present, table it until you can get the right people in the room.

Design a regular meeting schedule during the Pilot and stick to it. Great communication is the key to greasing the wheels of your new system. You only have 90 days for the entire Program and 40 days for the Pilot to get this system up and running. The more your team realizes that you're making the success of this system a priority, the more you'll have their support.

Congratulations! We're ready to go on to the next phase.

> **During Improve You Will:**
>
> ⦿ Create Your Pilot Checklists
>
> ⦿ Begin the Pilot
>
> ⦿ Begin Capturing Lessons Learned
>
> ⦿ Decide How You Will Measure Success

Welcome to Improve. By the time you have completed this phase you will be done or nearly done with the Pilot and ready to measure the effectiveness of your facility's new Notification Tracking System.

The Pilot is a specific period of time that your ED staff will begin using the Seven Steps program on the patient care floor. During and after the pilot, you and your Trauma Notification Manager will periodically meet with the Notification Team to measure the results, assess the success of the pilot and tweak anything that needs adjusting before the program is adopted and becomes policy.

Pilot Checklist

Is the Notification Tracking System Notebook set up and ready to go?

• Are the hand out documents that the Notification Team will receive prepared? Have you and the training and communications coordinator agreed upon when and where they will be distributed?

• Have the Notification Team and any allied department heads read an overview of the Seven Steps System?

• Is your management team on board with changes and pilot?

• Are all the Team's tools available and easy for them to find in the Emergency Department?

• Is the Notification Tracking System Notebook in its final location?

> o Does it contain all necessary reference materials and tools including:
>
> > • A Sample Patient Tracking Sheet and blank tracking sheets?
> >
> > • Definitions of Notification Team Roles and Responsibilities?
> >
> > • The Seven Steps?
> >
> > • Your Facility's Notification Work Flow?
> >
> > • Your Notification Policies (if applicable)?
> >
> > • Copies of Tip Sheets for Locating Emergency Contact Information, John Doe identification, or specialty notifications like pediatric, or Alzheimer's patients.
>
> o If you have notification reference material that doesn't fit in the Notebook, does the team know where to find it?
>
> o Is there a list of Notification Team Members and their pager numbers in the Tracking Notebook for quick identification when they are needed?
>
> o Are Patient Tracking Worksheets available for Assessors in triage or any other area where they perform initial patient assessments?

• If you are using an electronic version of the worksheet for a computer based charting system, make sure that it works correctly, and that your Team knows how to located it in the chart and how to use it.

• Does the team know who to contact with any questions, procedural problems or suggestions?

• Have you communicated your management routines and does everyone know when group meetings will take place?

• Does your Program Coordinator, TPM and your Follow Up team members know how to track notification and patient satisfaction results? (if you have decided to track them)

• Do you have a mechanism for gathering success stories during the pilot, or gathering different types of patients/notifications to discuss at group meetings.

• Have you discussed the Pilot with trauma managers, ED nurses and physicians? You should let them know that the Pilot is taking place and that it might take a few extra minutes for the Notification Team members to complete their work, as they focus on notifications, and break in the new system

• Do you have ways to engage your Notification Team and make them excited about the Notification Program? Consider doing incentives, or having recognitions for team members that do an outstanding job.

Measuring Results

Even though delighting patients and bringing families together during emergencies is satisfying in itself, we all know that hospitals are basically businesses. And businesses are concerned most of all, about the bottom line.

Results.

But results mean different things to different facilities. Possible positive results from implementing the Notification Tracking System could mean:

> • A reduction in the time it takes to identify a patient's emergency contacts, make the notification call and get the next of kin on site.

> • Higher patient satisfaction scores on the next facility survey.

> • Reducing liability by having all of your team's efforts to locate and notify a patient's next of kin documented in the patient record.

> • Reducing liability by obtaining the patient's full medical history from his family more quickly. Using a patient's actual history as a factor in their care, greatly reduces the likelihood of medical malpractice and drug interactions etc that can occur when physicians don't know a patient's history. Having patient's families on scene to give informed consent on procedures also reduces the likelihood of patient's families suing the hospital if the procedures go wrong..

> •A reduction in your ED staff workload.

So the goal with measuring results is gathering the right information and reporting them in a way that is meaningful, for your facility.

For the results to be meaningful, they need to be in line with your facility's goals and values. Go over the specific goals that your management team hopes to gain from the Pilot and the execution of the Notification Program in your facility, and enter them on the Measuring Results Tab of your Program Workbook. Then enter a few notes on the current state, the target state that you are seeking and if possible a measureable goal.

For example, if your goal is to reduce the time it takes to notify a patient's next of kin, the entry would look like this:

Goal	Current State	Target State	How Will Goal Be Measured?	Date
Reducing the time it takes for patient notifications to occur	6 hours for the first call to be made	2 hours for the first call to be made	When 80% or more of the Chart Worksheets document that the notifications have taken place in 2 hours or less	By June 30

You can set and measure as many overall goals as you like, but try to choose just a few goals that are important, yet easy to obtain. You're changing not only a process, but the habits of an entire team of people, so keep it simple. You can always add other goals and tweak systems or procedures that still need to be changed, once the Notification Program, becomes a permanent process.

Giving a measureable set of goals and quantifying their success, also gives you documentation that you can take to management to show them that your Pilot and Notification Program is working. In today's environment adding to your company's success certainly can't hurt!

And once you begin to see the successes, don't forget to recognize your Notification Team and your Program Team for their amazing work. Schedule a nice celebration in the cafeteria or put their photos in the hospital newsletter. Let your team know that they are appreciated. You should also elicit as many patient success and satisfaction stories as possible. If you can, add a question on to the next satisfaction survey addressing notifications and asking the patients and their families if they feel everything was done to reunite them together after an accident, trauma or serious illness. You can use those stories as a part of your success documentation and as a part of your facility's upcoming advertising or PR campaigns.

Lessons Learned

There is a tab on your Program Workbook called Lessons Learned. It captures everything that you and your team discover, learn or swear never to do again, during the Pilot and the execution of the Notification Program. Identifying the lessons and their remedy as it appears, will not only help you and your team perform notifications more effectively, but will help your facility the next time you undertake a new program or set of procedures. It's a teaching aid, a memory jogger and a way to record history so you aren't doomed to repeat it next time around. So make sure that your team knows where to send the lessons they discover along the way – either by email, a formal spreadsheet, or a phone call, with details that your Program Coordinator can enter into the Notification Workbook.

And Now... On To The Pilot

Once everything is ready to go, do the Program Kick Off and get the Pilot started.

The first morning the new system will be used, the Notification Program Manager and Trauma Notification Manager should be on hand in the Emergency Department, or at least very reachable by page or phone, to make sure everything goes well. Keep tabs on things for the first week and be visible. The last thing you want, is for your new team to be frustrated because no one is available to address questions or problems.

Since the Pilot only lasts 40 days, you and your team will have to work hard to ensure all the kinks are worked out before moving on to the execution phase of the program.

But don't worry. You're prepared, your team is prepared and this Pilot is going to go extremely well. We'll let you get back to work and meet you in the next phase – Control.

During Control You Will:

⊙ **Finalize Lessons Learned**

⊙ **Fine Tune Your Workflow and Chart Worksheet**

⊙ **Finalize Your Success Documentation**

⊙ **Grab Stories and Experiences that you can use for Testimonials**

⊙ **Turn the program over to the TNM to make it permanent policy in the ED.**

The Pilot is nearing its end and by now you have a good idea of its success and a handle on any problems that occurred.

How did it go? Are you happy with its success?

This is a great time to schedule a meeting of your Program Team and the Notification Team. Take about an hour or two to get everyone's feedback. If you're not getting a lot of conversation right off, the bat, try discussing a few of the lessons learned from your Program Worksheet or some interesting notifications from the Patient Tracking Worksheets. Have your Program Coordinator and your Training and Communication Coordinators note everyone's assessment of each part of the program. Here are a few questions to get you started:

• How well did the workflow function when you were making notifications?

• Were there any bottlenecks, or areas that didn't flow well?

• Were you able to find the information you needed to make notifications or identifications more easily than you did, before the Pilot?

• Is there anything about the system that just simply doesn't work?

• Is there anything that you would change about it?

• Our team has three specific team members per shift to handle notifications? Are three team members enough? Too many?

• Were you able to locate the staff members you needed, during weekends or in the middle of the night?

•Did you have any positive feedback from patients about the notification process?

•Any negative feedback from patients about the notification process?

•Did you have any positive feedback from other hospital staff members about the notification process?

•Any negative feedback from other hospital staff members about the notification process?

•Are there any other areas that we need to address before we make using the Notification System a permanent policy in the ED?

While you have everyone in the meeting, take out your Workflow(s) and Patient Tracking Worksheets and go over them with the team. If any problems or suggestions arise address them and make any necessary changes on the spot.

For the Follow Up people you'll also need to know what feedback they've heard from patients or their families during follow up calls or visits. If your Follow Up people have positive stories or outcomes to share, make sure that they are recorded in your Notification Workbook, for later use in your Program's success story or management updates. If they have any negative stories or experiences, use this forum to discuss what went wrong and what can be done in the future to prevent a negative outcome.

In the week or two between the official end of the pilot and the official adoption of the Notification System as permanent policy in your ED, continue to have your Notification Team perform the new workflow. But take the opportunity examine any problems that occurred or changes that need to be made, with your team, before the policy becomes a regulation in the ED.

Once anything that arose is addressed, turn the day to day management of the Seven Steps Notification System, over to the Trauma Notification Manager and add the workflow(s) and Patient Tracking Worksheet(s) your department is now using, to your facility's official notification policies.

You should follow the new system closely for about six months to make sure that the workflow and successes are maintained and that the system is second nature to the Notification Team. Ensure that the Tracking Notebook is being maintained as well and that all of the tools and reference materials are being updated and left in the notebook, where everyone can find them.

When you are certain that the system is a part of the culture in the ED, convene your Notification Program team one last time to go over your Program Workbook. Add anything additional that isn't already in there like, additional Lessons Learned, more patient or team member success stories, further communications or training plans. Complete any open items on your Measuring Improvement list, along with the date each goal was met and notes about its successful completion.

Congratulations you've done it!

Your patients are safer than ever and receiving the treatment they deserve with their medical history and specific needs in mind. You also have a system to document every notification as it happens, you've reduced your facility's liability in at least two areas and you've lightened the workload of your Emergency Department.

We'd love to hear from you. Please take a moment to share your success stories, comments and suggestions with us at webmaster1@nokep.org.

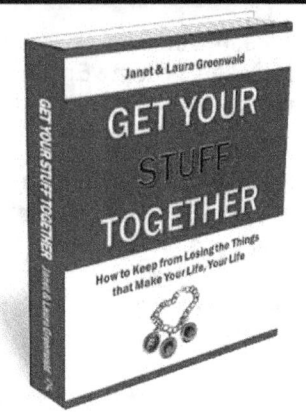

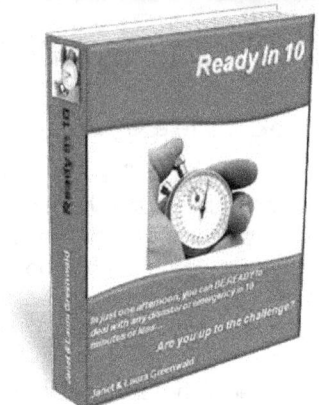

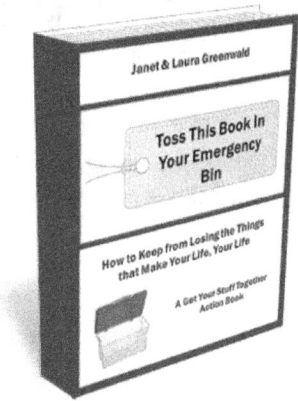

Get Your Stuff Together

Learn how to keep everything that's important to you, safe, sound and accessible, from family photos, vital documents and music, to videos, computer files & contacts.

Ready In 10

Are you totally unprepared for a disaster? Learn how to be able to grab everything you need -- necessities, keepsakes, vital information -- and evacuate in less than ten minutes.

Toss This Book In Your Emergency Bin

Have you ever wondered what to put in your Emergency Bin? The book puts all the information and plans you and your family need right at your fingertips.

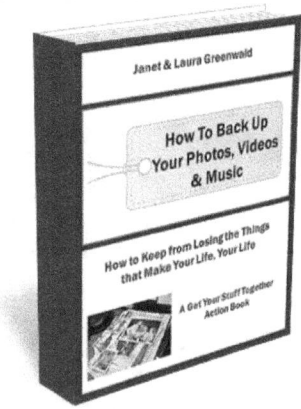

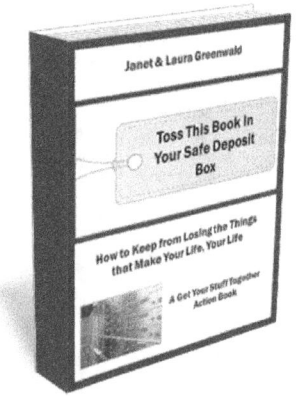

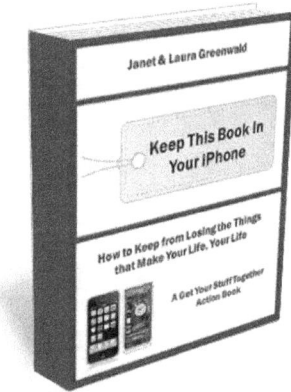

How To Back Up Your Photos, Videos & Music

Learn quick, easy steps to back up your print/digital photos, home movies, cassettes, vinyl albums and archive them in multiple, disaster proof locations.

Toss This Book In Your Safe Deposit Box

Take safety one step further by keeping all of your vital information, documents and keepsakes in two or more secure locations away from home.

Keep This Book In Your iPhone

All of the information & tools you need to turn your iPhone, Android or Smartphone into a mobile command center.

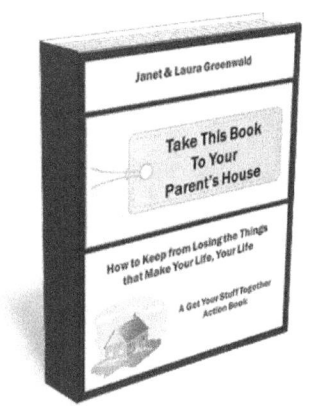

Take This Book To Your Parent's House

No one will forget the Superstorm Sandy footage of families searching through the wreckage of their homes only to find their cherished pictures and memories completely ruined. Don't let this tragedy happen to YOUR parents. Learn how to help them back up their photos, videos & keepsakes, information, medical history and vital documents.

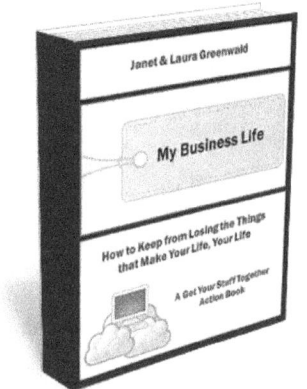

My Business Life

If you're an entrepreneur, you know what it takes to run a business. You have to wear many hats & the amount of information in your head is astounding. But what if you want to go to on vacation, or if you're sidelined due to injury or illness? With My Business Life, you'll have a place to record all of the information it takes to keep your business running.

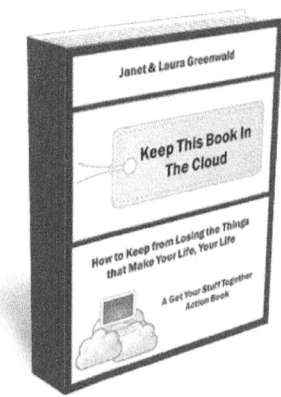

Keep This Book In The Cloud

You're savvy enough to know that it's not smart to only have your data and vital information in one location. But do you know how to back up that information and where to put it for safekeeping? And what if an emergency or disaster strikes while you're away from home? The book puts all the information and plans you and your family need right at your fingertips.

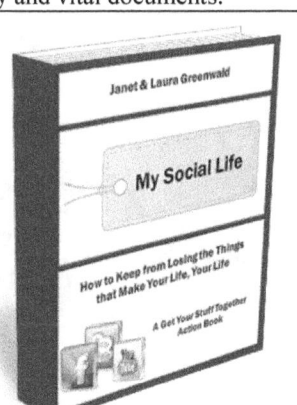

My Social Life

Finally! A place to record all of your social media accounts and passwords, putting your social life where it belongs. At your fingertips.

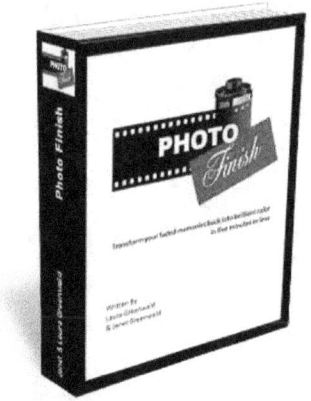

Photo Finish

Transform your faded photos back into brilliant color in five minutes or less. No more time, energy or effort. Just great results in five simple steps.

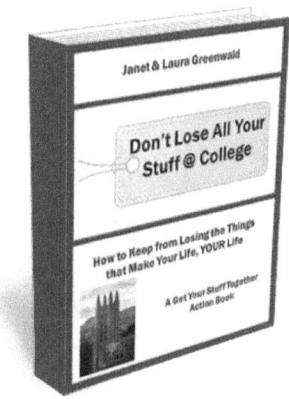

Don't Lose All Your Stuff At College

In one afternoon, your college student will learn the tools and resources he or she needs, to be safe and to stay safe.

Do yourself a favor. Get copies for yourself, copies for your best friend and copies for the people you love.

Bulk pricing and customization also available. www.getyourstufftogether.com

About The Authors

Janet and Laura Greenwald are one of the only mother and daughter screenwriting teams in the entertainment industry. They are authors of "Ready In 10," creators of the Ready In 10 downloadable Get Ready Kit and writers of original, one-hour dramas and screenplays including "Without Consent".

The Greenwalds were introduced to disaster preparedness the hard way, when a jumbo-jet crashed across the street from their home. After a few floods, earthquakes and a horrendous medical catastrophe that took the life of their mother/grandmother, Elaine Sullivan, they created three health care laws in California and Illinois, founded the Next of Kin Education Project and created Notify In 7, a nationally recognized next of kin training program for hospitals. When they found that so many other families had gone through similar experiences as they had, they decided to share their story to keep other families from having to live through the same medical nightmare. The result was "Without Consent," a screenplay for a feature film that is already attracting attention from actors and producers.

After seeing hundreds of thousands of people suffering so much loss during the last few years -- from Hurricane Katrina, to the Japan, Chile and Haiti earthquakes, along with countless tornadoes and floods – the Greenwalds decided to use the knowledge and tools they had gained to teach families how to be ready to deal with any disaster or emergency in 10 minutes. The result was "Ready In 10," one of the only downloadable disaster preparedness kits in existence.

"Ready In 10" and "Get Your Stuff Together" contain ten steps that can easily be completed in one afternoon. It is specially designed to help people get through a disaster or emergency with their loved ones, vital documents and keepsakes intact. In other words they won't just survive a disaster, they'll be able to pick up their lives and go on as quickly as possible.

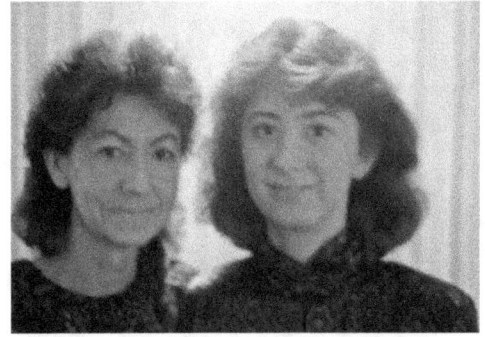